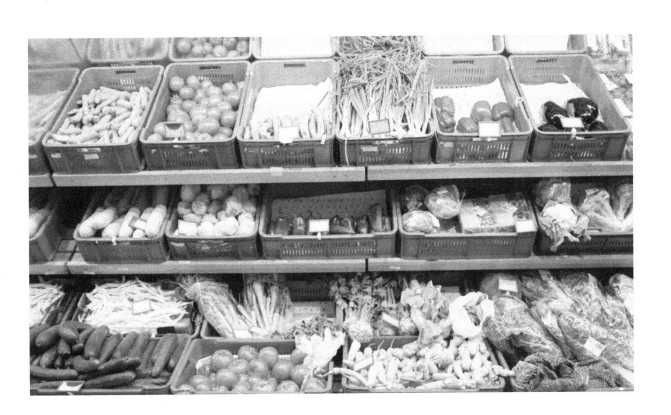

PLANT-BASED DIET 2021

THE IDEAL GUIDE TO START EATING WITH A PLANT-BASED DIET TO LOSE WEIGHT, LIVE BETTER AND STAY FIT. RESTORE YOUR HEALTH AND KEEP YOUR SUGAR LEVELS AND BLOOD PRESSURE DOWN

Table of contents

Contents

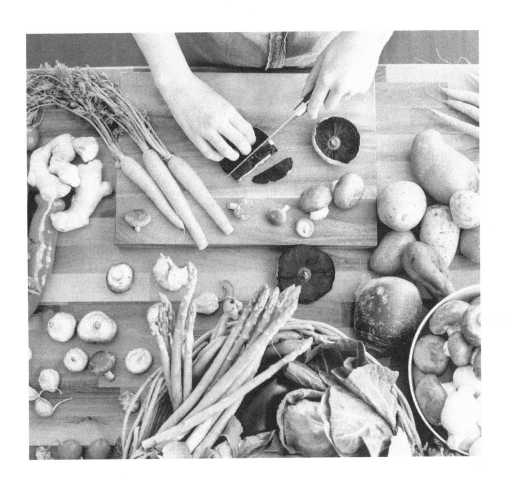

PLANT-BASED DIET

INTRODUCTION

Plant-based or whole plant eating center on nourishments basically from plants. This incorporates fruits and vegetables, yet also nuts, seeds, oils, entire grains, vegetables, and beans. It doesn't imply that you are vegetarian or vegan and never eat meat or dairy. Or maybe, you are proportionately picking a higher amount of your nourishments from plant sources.

Plant-based weight control plans offer all the essential protein, fats, carbohydrates, nutrients, and minerals for ideal wellbeing, and are regularly higher in fiber and phytonutrients. Notwithstanding, a few vegans may need to include an enhancement (explicitly nutrient B12) to guarantee they get every one of the nutrients required.

There is no reasonable meaning of what comprises an entire nourishments, plant-based eating regimen (WFPB diet). The WFPB diet isn't a set eating regimen — it's to a higher degree a way of life. This is because plant-based eating regimens can shift enormously, relying upon the degree to which an individual incorporates creature items in their eating regimen.

Regardless, the essential standards of an entire nourishments, plant-based diet are as per the following:

- Emphasizes full, negligibly handled nourishments.

- Limits or stays away from creature items.

- Focuses on plants, including vegetables, fruits, entire grains, vegetables, seeds, and nuts, which should make up most of what you eat.

- Excludes refined nourishments, as included sugars, white flour, and handled oils.

- Pays extraordinary consideration regarding nourishment quality, with numerous advocates of the WFPB diet advancing privately sourced, natural nourishment at whatever point conceivable.

Hence, this eating regimen is regularly mistaken for vegan or vegetarian eats less. However, albeit comparable here and there, these weight control plans are not the equivalent.

Individuals who pursue vegan diets go without expending any creature items, including dairy, meat, poultry, fish, eggs, and nectar. Vegetarians bar all meat and poultry from their eating regimens, yet a few vegetarians eat eggs, fish, or dairy. The WFPB diet, then again, is progressively adaptable. Devotees eat for the most part plants. However, creature items aren't off cutoff points. While one individual after a WFPB diet may eat no creature items, another may eat limited quantities of eggs, poultry, fish, meat, or dairy.

In this digital book, you will comprehend the significance of entire plant-based eating routine, the overview and the impact of plant put together diets with respect to our body, the helpful properties of plant-based nourishment, the a month plant-based meal plan, the significant recipes to watch out for when considering plant-based meal, for example, the morning meal recipes, the smoothies recipes, the soup recipes for plant found weight control plans, the plates of mixed greens recipes, the primary dishes and sauce recipes, the deserts and beverages.

WHAT IS A PLANT-BASED DIET

A plant-based diet is an eating routine focused after eating plants, with practically no creature items. Nourishment that is a piece of a plant-based eating regimen incorporates fruits, vegetables, grains, vegetables, nuts, and seeds.

The advantages of eating a plant-based eating routine are interminable. It can have an assortment of positive wellbeing consequences for people, it harms fewer creatures than a standard American eating regimen, and it has a much lower ecological impression.

What Does A Plant-Based Diet Mean?

Natural, non-GMO, nearby, plant-based. It appears to be each day there's new nourishment and diet marks to learn on the off chance that you need to comprehend where your food is coming from or how it impacts your wellbeing.

In any case, a plant-based eating regimen isn't incredible for your wellbeing, however extraordinary for the life span of the planet. Be that as it may, not at all like stylish eating regimens that endeavor to confine what you eat seriously or the amount you eat, there's not so much a reasonable meaning of what essentially establishes a plant-based eating routine. That is because plant-based eating isn't just about what you placed in your body; it's about your general way of life.

Plant-put together diets all depend concerning the degree to which an individual incorporates creature items in their standard dietary patterns. Before you start tossing everything out of your icebox, how about we separate the nuts and bolts of eating a plant-based eating regimen.

What Is a Whole Food Plant-Based Diet?

Numerous individuals who pursue a plant-based diet for wellbeing reasons attempt to adhere to a whole nourishments plant-based (WFPB) diet, which spotlights on eating nourishments in their entire structure, as they show up in nature. Somebody eating a WFPB food may likewise restrain their utilization of prepared or refined nourishments, for example, oil, refined sugar, white flour, and bundled snacks made with synthetics.

What Is Veganism?

Veganism is a way of life that looks to bar the utilization of creatures, however much as could reasonably be expected. Going vegan is generally a choice one makes dependent on moral reasons, in the wake of finding out about the creature farming industry's poor treatment of animals, just as the business's high ecological effect.

Does Plant-Based Mean Vegan?

The terms vegan and plant-based are frequently utilized reciprocally — and keeping in mind that the two times are fundamentally the same as there are a couple of contrasts.

A vegan eats a plant-based diet — yet that is just a single some portion of veganism. Notwithstanding nourishments like dairy, meat, fish, eggs, and nectar, vegans additionally maintain a strategic distance from creature determined added substances like gelatin and lanolin. Furthermore, vegans expand their conviction that animals ought not to be utilized by people past what's on their plates, running from beautifying agents to family cleaning items to dress to furniture.

Alternately, somebody who eats a plant-based eating routine isn't a vegan. The inspiration driving veganism is the creatures and regularly the Earth, while the inspiration driving a plant-based eating routine is generally wellbeing or weight loss (however, that is not an immovable standard). Hence, individuals following a plant-based eating routine may treat it like only that — an eating regimen — and in this way every so often eat creature items; they may eat nourishments made with creature determined added substances; they may likewise still purchase dress, furnishings or different things produced using creature materials, for example, cowhide, fleece, and hide; and they may purchase individual cleanliness items that were tried on creatures.

All things considered, eating a plant-based diet with wellbeing as your inspiration is as yet an extraordinary thing. Not exclusively can eating for the most part plants help forestall and invert sickness, help in weight loss, and streamline wellbeing, yet you'll additionally appreciate the positive reactions of helping your ecological impression, and you'll hurt fewer creatures.

The basics of a plant-based eating routine include:

- Eating insignificantly prepared, negligibly foul entire nourishments and plants. Think vegetables, fruits, whole grains, vegetables, seeds, and nuts.

- Limiting or keeping away from creature items like meat, dairy items, eggs, and fish, and instead picking supportable protein options like beans, tofu, tempeh, and so on.

- Avoiding profoundly refined nourishments like blanched flour, refined sugar, trans-fats, oil, and nourishment synthetic substances.

Not at all like vegan and vegetarian eats less, a plant-based eating regimen offers somewhat more adaptability. Even though it's urged to confine the measure of animal-based items one devours, it doesn't out and out limit them. So while some may expel dairy items from their eating routine totally, others may, in any case, eat eggs at early lunch or choose it doesn't trouble them if their morning latte has whole milk.

Load up on reliable minimal effort staples. Cut back on your meat consumption. Pick natural, unfenced chicken, meat, and eggs when you choose to eat them. Know your names, discover where your meat and produce are sourced from and have some good times exploring different avenues regarding new recipes. These are on the whole essential pieces of eating an eating routine that accentuations entire nourishment, plant-based meals.

Not every person is prepared to make the bounce into plant-based destroying the right, and that is alright. Rather than promptly focusing on an eating regimen you aren't acquainted with, take a stab at supplanting a couple of meals during the time with vegetarian alternatives.

Why You Need to Cut Back On Processed and Animal-Based Products

You've likely heard on numerous occasions that prepared food is terrible for you. "Maintain a strategic distance from additives; stay away from prepared foods"; be that as it may, nobody ever truly gives you any right or generous data on why you ought to keep away from them and why they are risky. So how about we separate it so you can completely comprehend why you ought to dodge these guilty parties. They have significant addictive properties. As people, we have a robust inclination to be dependent on specific foods. However, the truth of the matter is that it's not so much our flaw. The entirety of the unfortunate eats we enjoy, every once in awhile, enact our cerebrums dopamine synapse. This makes the cerebrum feel "great," yet just for a short period. This additionally makes a fixation propensity; that is the reason somebody will consistently wind up returning for another sweet treat, although they needn't bother with it. You can maintain a distance from this by expelling that upgrade all things considered.

They are stacked sugar and high fructose corn syrup. Prepared and animal-based items are stacked with sugars and high fructose corn syrup, which have near-zero healthy benefits. An ever-increasing number of studies are currently demonstrating what many individuals speculated up and down; that hereditarily adjusted foods because gut irritation, which like this, makes it harder for the body to retain fundamental supplements. The drawback of your body neglecting to preserve essential supplements, from muscle misfortune appropriately and mind mist to fat increase, can't be focused on enough.

They are stacked with refined starches processed foods, and abased items are stacked with refined carbs. Indeed, your body needs carbs to give vitality to run body capacities. In any case, refining carbs takes out the essential supplements; in the manner in which that refining entire grains decrease the whole grain part. What you are left within the wake of refining is what's alluded to as "unfilled" carbs. These can negatively affect your digestion by spiking your glucose and insulin levels.

They are stacked with fake fixings. At the point when your body is expending counterfeit fixings, and it regards them as an outside article. They become an intruder. Your body isn't accustomed to perceiving things like sucralose or these artificial sugars. Along these lines, your body does what it specializes in. It triggers an insusceptible reaction, which brings down your obstruction, making you defenseless against infections. The concentration and vitality spent by your body in ensuring your insusceptible framework could make some way or another be occupied somewhere else.

They contain parts that reason a hyper reward sense in your body. This means they contain segments like monosodium glutamate (MSG), portions of high fructose corn syrup, and specific colors that can cut addictive properties. They animate your body to receive a reward in return. MSG, for example, is in a great deal of pre-bundled baked goods. What this does is that it invigorates your taste buds to appreciate the taste. It becomes mental just by how your mind speaks with your taste buds. This reward-based framework makes your body need increasingly more of it putting.

You at extreme danger of caloric overconsumption. Shouldn't something be said about creature protein? Regularly the expression "low quality" is tossed around to plant proteins allude to since they will, in general, have lower measures of essential amino acids contrasted with creature protein. What the vast majority don't understand is that increasingly fundamental amino acids can be very harming to your wellbeing. Along these lines, how about we rapidly clarify how.

Creature Protein Lacks Fiber In their mission to load up on progressively creature protein, and a great many people wind up uprooting the plant protein that they previously had. This is awful because, dissimilar to plant protein, a creature protein regularly needs fiber, cell reinforcements, and phytonutrients. Fiber lack is very reasonable crosswise over various networks and social orders on the planet. For example, as per the Institute of Medicine, the average grown-up expends pretty much 15 grams of fiber for each day against the prescribed 38 grams. The absence of satisfactory dietary fiber admission is related to an expanded danger of colon and bosom malignant growths, just as Crohn's ailment, coronary illness, and stoppage. Creature protein causes a spike in IGF-1 IGF-1 is the hormone-insulin-like development factor-1.

It invigorates cell division and development, which may seem like something to be thankful for. However, it likewise animates the development of malignant growth cells. Higher blood levels of IGF-1 are accordingly connected with expanded disease dangers, harm, and expansion. Creature protein causes an increase in Phosphorus Animal protein contains elevated levels of phosphorus. Our bodies standardize the significant levels of phosphorus by discharging a hormone called fibroblast development factor 23 (FGF23). This hormone is destructive to our veins,

On account of an examination titled "Circling Fibroblast Growth Factor 23 Is Associated with Angiographic Severity and Extent of Coronary Artery Disease,". FGF23 has additionally been found to cause sporadic expansion of cardiovascular muscles – a hazard factor for cardiovascular breakdown and even passing in extreme cases. Given every one of the issues, the "excellent" part of creature protein may be all the more fittingly depicted as "high chance." In contrast to caffeine, which you will encounter withdrawal once you cut it off totally, prepared foods can be cut off immediately. Maybe the one thing that you'll miss is the comfort of not setting up each dinner without any preparation.

Plant-Based Diet versus Veggie lover It is fundamental for individuals to confuse a vegetarian diet with a plant-based diet or the other way around. Although the two diets share likenesses, they are not the equivalent. So how about we separate it genuine speedy. Veggie lover A vegetarian diet is one that contains no abased items.
This incorporates meat, dairy, eggs just as determined items or fixings, for example, nectar. Somebody who depicts themselves as a vegetarian extends this point of view into their regular day to day existence. This means they don't utilize or advance the utilization of garments, shoes, embellishments, cleansers, and cosmetics that have been made using a material that originates from creatures. Models here incorporate fleece, beeswax, calfskin, gelatin, silk, and lanolin. The inspiration for individuals to lead a veganism way of life frequently comes from a craving to hold fast and battle against creature abuse and poor moral treatment of creatures to advance well as basic entitlements.

Plant-Based Diet An entire food plant-based diet, then again, shares comparability with veganism as it likewise doesn't advance dietary utilization of animal-based items. This incorporates dairy, meat, and eggs. What's more, is that not healthy for the vegetarian diet, prepared foods, white flour, oils, and refined sugars are not part of the menu.
The thought here is to make a diet out of insignificantly handled to natural organic products, veggies, entire grains, nuts, seeds, and vegetables. Along these lines, there will be NO Oreo treats for you. Whole food plant-based diet supporters are regularly determined by the medical advantages it brings. It is a diet that has next to no to do with limiting calories or checking.
Macros yet generally to do with anticipating and turning around diseases.

HISTORICAL ORIGINS OF THIS DIET

A plant-based diet is an eating routine comprising for the most part or altogether of nourishments got from plants, including vegetables, grains, nuts, seeds, vegetables and fruits, and with few or no creature products. A plant-based diet isn't vegetarian.

The utilization of the expressed plant-based diet has changed after some time, and models can be found of the expression "plant-based diet," is used to allude to vegan consumes fewer calories, which contain no nourishment from animals sources. To vegetarian eats less, which includes eggs and dairy yet no meat, and to eats fewer carbs with fluctuating measures of creature-based nourishments, for example, semi-vegetarian eats fewer carbs which contain modest quantities of meat.

Well-arranged plant diets bolster wellbeing and are proper all through life, including pregnancy, lactation, adolescence, adulthood, and for competitors.

Very few sources utilize the expression plant-based diet to allude to diets including changing degrees of creature items, characterizing "plant-based abstains from food" as, "slims down that incorporate liberal measures of plant nourishments and restricted measures of creature nourishments", and as diets "wealthy in an assortment of vegetables and fruits, vegetables, and insignificantly prepared boring staple nourishments and constraining red meat utilization, if red meat is eaten at all".

Others draw a differentiation between "plant-based" and "plant-only."

In different sources, "plant-based eating regimen" has been utilized to allude to:

• Veganism: diet of vegetables, vegetables, fruit, grains, nuts, and seeds, yet no nourishment from creature sources.[8]

✓ Fruitarianism: vegan diet comprising fundamentally of fruit.
✓ Raw veganism: vegan diet in which nourishment is uncooked and once in a while dehydrated.
✓

• Vegetarianism: diet of vegetables, vegetables, fruit, nuts, and grains, that may incorporate eggs and dairy, however no meat.

✓ Ovo-lacto vegetarianism: incorporates dairy and eggs
✓ Ovo vegetarianism: incorporates eggs however no dairy
✓ Lacto vegetarianism: incorporates dairy however no eggs

Despite the fact that herbivory (dependence on diet completely of plants) was for some time thought to be a Mesozoic wonder, proof of it is found when the fossils which could show it. Inside under 20 million years after the primary land plants advanced, plants were being devoured by arthropods.[13] Herbivory among four-limbed earthbound vertebrates, the tetrapods created in the Late Carboniferous (307 - 299 million years ago).[14] Early tetrapods were enormous land and/or water capable piscivores. While creatures of land and water kept on benefiting from fish and creepy crawlies, a few reptiles started investigating two new nourishment types: the tetrapods (carnivory) and plants (herbivory).[14]

Carnivory was a characteristic transition from insectivory for medium and enormous tetrapods, requiring negligible adjustment. Interestingly, a mind boggling set of adjustments was vital for benefiting from exceptionally stringy plant materials.[14]

Present day herbivores and gentle omnivory

Frequently, for the most part herbivorous animals will eat little amounts of creature based nourishment when it gets accessible. If this is insignificant more often than not, omnivorous or herbivorous flying creatures, for example, sparrows, regularly will bolster their chicks creepy crawlies while nourishment is most required for growth.

On close assessment apparently nectar-encouraging flying creatures, for example, sunbirds depend on the ants and different creepy crawlies that they find in blooms, not for a more extravagant inventory of protein, yet for fundamental nutrients, for example, Vitamin B12 that are missing from nectar. So also, monkeys of numerous species eat rancid fruit, now and again in clear inclination to sound fruit.[16] When to allude to such creatures as omnivorous or something else, is an issue of setting and accentuation, instead of definition.

The ascent of the vegetarian and, all the more as of late, the vegan diet is commonly seen to be another wonder. Along these lines, as well, is their relationship with contemporary dynamic thoughts, governmental issues and ways of life. Yet, plant-based weight control plans have profound verifiable roots, and a longstanding association with the political left.

From the hour of the 1789 French upset, when radical thoughts were clearing Europe, a political, moral vegetarianism has developed close by the British left. Pushed by significant figures from the writer Percy Shelley to dramatist George Bernard Shaw – just as a lot more in spearheading radical associations and networks – contemporary composing exhibits how a plant-based eating routine created as a component of left-wing belief system, activism and character.

Understand more: Should veganism get a similar legitimate insurance as a religion?

During the 1790s, a few British radicals received vegetarianism as a major aspect of their more extensive endeavors to upset the current universality. Affected by rationalist Jean-Jacques Rousseau's standards with respect to a "characteristic state" of opportunity, harmony and balance, individuals, for example, the Anglo-Jacobin progressive John Oswald, the extreme researcher Joseph Ritson, and the distributer George Nicholson advanced the eating routine as a focal component of their extensive contentions for equity and cooperation.

The eating regimen had a huge nearness in the Romantic time frame, particularly inside the hover of Percy and Mary Shelley. Percy Shelley composed two articles supporting vegetarianism, one of which – A Vindication of Natural Diet (1813) – was attached to his persuasive progressive ballad Queen Mab.

Sovereign Mab anticipated a "heaven of harmony", a condition of partnership between every living being, in which "man has lost/His awful privilege" to deny others of life. Delineating a straightforward, satisfying presence drove in amicability with nature, it showed a world "equivalent, unclassed, tribeless, and nationless", without unnecessary clash and division.

Morals and nature

Vegetarianism proceeded with its relationship with the incipient left all through the right on time to mid-nineteenth century and turned into a typical component of communism constantly close. Albeit generally grounded in morals, contentions were additionally created about its wellbeing and biological advantages. These focused on the ecological weights of meat generation, and tried to counter a developing mechanical industrialist society of harming over-utilization.

Understand progressively: Going veggie would cut worldwide nourishment emanations by 66% and spare a great many lives – new investigation

Veganism was frequently recognized as the perfect, including by the blade de-siècle communist, helpful campaigner and spearheading basic entitlements advocate Henry Salt. Impacted by the thoughts of Shelley, just as the anarcho-socialism of Peter Kropotkin and the transformative hypotheses of Alfred Russell Wallace – both of whom focused on the significance of participation, rather than rivalry, in nature – Salt laid out a vegetarian-liberal standpoint average of the period.

Contending that all types of abuse were interconnected, he upheld "not either accommodating change, yet every one of them" at the same time, for it was anything but a solitary explicit indication, however the root "infection" – society's basic ethic – that necessary treatment.

Salt distinguished this as one of narrow minded abuse, thus pushed a steady standard of empathy to restrict it, battling for the reasons for communism, ladies' freedom, pacifism, vegetarianism and basic entitlements. All were, he attested, "indistinguishably associated" and none could "be completely acknowledged alone". He consequently advanced the expansion of "empathy, love and equity" to "each living animal", as a component of a far reaching moral belief. He composed:

Viciousness generates savagery

Since this commencement, vegetarianism has been most connected with increasingly all-encompassing types of radical idea – those which look past financial aspects to concentrate on the individual, good and profound parts of communism. These "elective" strands were especially prevalent in the nineteenth century. Commonly named "libertarian" or "moral", they accentuated the interconnection of individual and cultural change, hostile to dictatorship and thoughts of sweeping freedom.

'The casualties of the pot and skillet went forward against the dictator man'. A bull conveys the warning surmounted by an improved cooking pot in this picture by the acclaimed communist craftsman, and vegetarian, Walter Crane (1911). Creator gave

Many received the vegetarian diet since they perceived that brutality towards different creatures, and meat eating specifically, was an integral part of the rough, exploitative society encompassing them. A general public, as portrayed by Salt, described by ruthless utilization and wherein people, especially the first class, turned out to be "truly man-eaters … eating up the fragile living creature and blood of the non-human creatures so firmly much the same as us, and in a roundabout way man-eaters, as living by the perspiration and drudge of the classes who do the diligent work of the world."

In the perspective on Salt and others, meat eating habituated savage practices and demeanors, disintegrated mankind's altruistic impulses, and undermined the very premise of a perfect tranquil, helpful society. To contradict meat eating was along these lines to challenge existing society, and to endeavor to change its fundamental ethic of abuse and predation to one of sympathy and participation.

Another method for being

Encapsulating all inclusive harmony and cooperation, vegetarianism spoke to another method for being. Consequently, its training by key figures in the historical backdrop of peacefulness, from Percy Shelley to Leo Tolstoy and Mahatma Gandhi, comes as meager astonishment.

Similarly, meat eating came to encapsulate a counter-type of this belief system, with meat utilization regularly connected with manly, battle ready and patriot governmental issues – as exemplified by the nineteenth century imagery encompassing John Bull, the devoted hamburger eating English everyman.

James Gillray's John Bull Taking a Luncheon. Bull regularly typified the meat-eating everyman. James Gillray through Wikimedia Commons

In this light, the eating regimen's specific appropriation by various pioneer women's activists and suffragettes, particularly the individuals who additionally distinguished as socialists, for example, Charlotte Despard and Isabella Ford and, in the US, Charlotte Perkins Gilman, served not just as a dismissal of the exploitative viciousness of an out of line social request, yet of man centric society itself.

Through the twentieth century, vegetarianism's relationship with the left proceeded, with various noticeable Labor MPs, including Fenner Brockway and Tony Benn, rehearsing the eating routine. Also, today, to purposely specify Jeremy Corbyn's vegetarianism is right around a prosaism.

Be that as it may, presently it is making strides among more youthful ages, as well. Against the scenery of the atmosphere emergency, and with a developing craving for another legislative issues of resilience, empathy and collaboration, which tries to destroy blinding obstructions and divisions, vegetarianism and veganism show up progressively pertinent.

WHAT YOU WILL BE EATING

Purposes behind Meal Planning
Plant-based meal arranging is somewhat more muddled first and foremost contrasted with simply preparing up irregular meals. Things being what they are, the reason the hell would it be a good idea for you to significantly trouble and teach yourself on the best way to meal plan appropriately? Indeed, it can offer you a greater number of advantages than you may suspect.

How might you like:

- A fluff-free week

- Less basic leadership and overthinking meals

- Easier shopping and a lower staple bill

- Effortlessly adhering to sound propensities.

- Easily meeting individual dietary needs.

- Trying new recipes

- Having an arrangement for your weight loss or weight gain

- Knowing what works best for you

- Keeping yourself responsible by having every one of the fixings and meals close by

Beginning Tips
Before we're getting directly into the vegan meat of the issue, there are a couple of tips to think about that can make your meal arranging venture significantly simpler, less startling, and considerably more energizing! We truly need you to succeed, and this implies you're getting a charge out of the procedure just as the outcomes here.

In this way, here are our top beginning tips:
Keep a nourishment diary to follow which meals you and your family loved just as how much exertion or time they require, so you know whether and when to incorporate them in your next meal plan.
Go for simple meals before all else, possibly only 3-4 fixings each. A model would be, beans, and broccoli, avocado. The nourishments don't require a lot of cooking abilities or time to prepare and can be cluster cooked effectively.
Talking about which, start to clump single cooking elements for quick is the meals. Get beans that can be eaten with rice, in a soup, a plate of mixed greens, or pureed and grains which can be utilized for sautés, servings of mixed greens, stews, bowls, or breakfast porridge.

Pay special mind to recipes you could go without much of a stretch twofold for remains to take to lunch like stew, soups, or bean burgers.

Plan meals you're now acquainted with, supplanting the creature-based nourishments with vegan partners like tofu cuts for chicken and pureed beans for cream cheddar.

Ask your accomplice or children what they might want to eat so everybody's content with what will be on the table.

Continue gathering recipes that look intriguing and attempt another one consistently when you have additional time. You can utilize the web for some motivation!

Additionally, keep a rundown of recipes that function admirably for yourself and your family so you can recall what to get ready for the following weeks.

At last, get imaginative with new blends and think outside about the container to keep things energizing! Soba noodle serving of mixed greens, anybody?

Picking your nourishment

There are lots of interesting points when picking the nourishments which you will incorporate into your meal plan. Once more, remember these to make the procedure increasingly charming and fun! Along these lines, for your plant-based meal arranging, ensure you.

-
- Go for the nourishments you effectively like before purchasing an enormous pack of Brussel's sprouts or rhubarb.

- Add assortment through various flavorings and flavours, for example, curry glue, paprika, Italian herbs, mustard, soy sauce, or BBQ sauce.

- Use what you have at home to set aside cash and abstain from squandering any nourishment.

- Keep a running rundown of what you need so you won't overlook anything and remain well-loaded

- Make a staple rundown to go out on the town to shop each week.

- Go for mass areas and occasional produce to set aside some cash.

- Design your meal plan to your taste, season, and what's least expensive to purchase in your general vicinity.

- Look out for solidified or pre-cut/pre-destroyed produce and canned vegetables to make your life simpler.

Next, we should stock up your kitchen! By what other means would you have the option to look over a decent assortment of delicious, solid, and flexible nourishments to use in your meal plan?

We're searching for filling staples, for example, rice, beans, millet, quinoa, lentils, entire grain pasta, potatoes, sweet potatoes, winter squash, and corn. For toppings and additional items, you can likewise get your top picks nuts and seeds.

Add new or solidified produce to these dull staples. It's good to have some verdant greens in the cooler, alongside tomatoes, cucumber, ringer pepper, cruciferous vegetables, zucchini, eggplant, and mushrooms. Pick what you like the most, and what's accessible to you! Solidified berries are constantly a decent choice, so are bananas, dates, apples, and oranges.

For our fixings and flavourings, we like having some soy milk (or other plant-based milk), soy yoghurt, mustard, ketchup, hot sauce, soy sauce, wholesome yeast, maple syrup, vinegar, lemon juice and a lot of flavors.

Additional tip: Have a consistent stockpile of snacks in the house, for example, natural product, nuts, and wafers!

We should Plan!

Since you've found out about probably the most significant establishments, we can get into the arranging it-hard and fast part. When thinking of an idea for a meal plan, we like to concentrate on the accompanying rules. Check whether your nourishment or meals are:

- Nutrient thick

- Low in included fat, salt and sugar

- Rich in fiber

- Filling and fulfilling

- Based on starches

- Adequate to meet your caloric and dietary needs

This may appear to be somewhat conceptual to you at present, so we needed to give you a clearer picture of what your meals ought to resemble.

Your morning meals could comprise of:

Starches

Oats, bread, oat, hash tans, hotcakes

Vegetables

Soy milk, soy yoghurt, tofu (for scramble), nutty spread

Natural product

New, dried, solidified, for example, berries, apples, bananas.

Nuts and Seeds

Flaxseeds, chia seeds, pecans, almond spread

Your lunches and suppers could comprise of:

Starches

Potatoes, pasta, rice, bread, couscous, bulgur, millet

Vegetables

Beans, lentils, tofu, soy milk, hummus, tempeh

Vegetables

Verdant greens, broccoli, chime pepper, zucchini, muhrooms

Additional items

Nuts, seeds, natural product, sauces, flavours, fixings

Concerning snacks, there are no fixed principles – do whatever it takes not to utilize this season of day to sneak some garbage or candy machine nourishment into your eating regimen. Some better thoughts are a new natural product, dried organic product, nuts, entire grain saltines, rice cakes, hummus, veggie sticks, cooked chickpeas, granola bars, sans oil popcorn, or just a few remains.

Some of you may think now: "Yet in what manner will I meet the majority of my wholesome needs if I don't generally follow my nourishment? Isn't that difficult on a plant-based eating regimen?" This next part is for you to teach yourself and facilitate your brain.

Supplements and nourishments to concentrate on
We need to begin by saying that an entire nourishments plant-based eating regimen is just about the most supplement thick diet you could think of. That being stated, there are still approaches to pass up a couple of basic ones if you don't concentrate on a pleasant assortment of nourishments. A few people like to eat a lot of natural products or starches, disregarding vegetables and seeds, for instance.

It's not simpler for individuals on an omnivorous eating regimen to meet the majority of their healthful needs since they generally get too little fibre, nutrients, and minerals while having an excessive amount of immersed fat and cholesterol. In this manner, everybody ought to design their eating regimen carefully!

Concerning a couple of supplements that are somewhat harder to jump on a plant-based eating routine, below best sources to go for and incorporate into your everyday diet. Pick at any rate one for every supplement:

• Calcium: strengthened soy milk, tofu, kale, broccoli, vegetables, sesame, entire wheat

• Iron: vegetables, tofu, tomato sauce, dull green vegetables, oats, quinoa, dark-coloured rice

• Zinc: pumpkin seeds, vegetables, entire grains, verdant green vegetables

• Omega-3: flaxseed, chia seeds, pecans, romaine lettuce

• Vitamin B12: supplements, strengthened nourishment

• Vitamin D: daylight, a few mushrooms, strengthened nourishments, supplements.

Parts and calories

You may, at present, be pondering about the amount to eat on a plant-based eating regimen. In case you're not mindful of your everyday prescribed vitality consumption, check your BMR and include your movement level utilizing a straightforward number cruncher. Most grown-ups need around at any rate 2000 calories for each day, which you shouldn't attempt to undermine excessively, in any event, when attempting to get more fit.
Plant-based nourishments, particularly when entire and natural, have a lower calorie thickness, which means you should eat bigger segments, and it will be significantly simpler to lose some weight because these food sources include considerably more mass.
If you wind up excessively stuffed or too hungry following a day of eating, make a note and modify the following day appropriately or at whatever point you're making your new meal plan. We can't reveal to you precisely the amount you have to eat, so please have your age, sex, activity level, a feeling of anxiety, and wellbeing status at the top of the priority list. We're advocates for eating instinctively, which means get something when you're eager and quit chewing when you're serenely full.
It's on you to choose what number of meals every day you'd like to eat and if you need to snack. Various things work for various individuals here. Regardless of if it's 2, 3, 4, or 5 little meals for every day – work with your inclinations and your timetable.

Altering for weight objectives

When changing your meal plan to your needs and objectives, we advise that you move your concentration starting with one nutrition class then onto the next and not to remove something. All entire plant-based nourishments are helpful to your wellbeing (insofar as you're not narrow-minded or susceptible to them) and can be eaten. We're working with the rule of calorie thickness here which you can use to either lose, gain, or keep up your weight while energizing your body with solid nourishments.

In case you're into weight picking up or lifting weights, centre more on entire flour items and vegetables just as nuts, seeds, and dried natural product to get enough calories. The equivalent goes for individuals with a little craving who battle with eating enough. You may likewise need to incorporate more smoothies and even squeezes into your eating regimen to expand your calories. Go simple on gigantic crude plates of mixed greens and vegetable stews since they offer just a couple of calories while including a ton of mass.

Similarly, in case you're into weight loss, centre on non-bland vegetables to go with your entire, flawless starches like potatoes or darker rice for lunch and supper. Try not to reduce the starches excessively, have around half vegetables and starches on your plate. Go simple on flour items and dried natural product, have the crisp organic product as a snack and attempt to eat a green serving of mixed greens each day. Likewise, keep away from included oils and lessen the measure of nuts and seeds you expend.

Is entire nourishment, plant-based eating routine, with organic products, vegetables, vegetables, nuts, and grains that come straightforwardly from nature? Following twenty years in the regular wellbeing industry, I realize that following a plant-based eating routine that is free of prepared and bundled nourishments — and including exercise and an inspirational demeanour — will present to you the best outcomes for your wellbeing and happiness.

I have attempted numerous weight control plans, including crude vegan, sans gluten, fruitarian, and plant-based Keto. At present, I pursue a plant-based eating routine, concentrating on entire natural nourishment. I accept that being excessively exacting in one's eating routine may prompt a few difficulties and even despair, so I pursue the 90/10 guideline, eating carefully plant-based 90 per cent of the time, with 10 per cent took into consideration the periodic utilization of crude goat or sheep cheddar, yet never meat or eggs. I additionally participate in discontinuous fasting, and obviously, customary exercise, contemplation, and enhancements to adjust my nourishment.

Brisk Tips to Start a Plant-Based Diet

A plant-based eating regimen underscores entire, natural vegetables, natural products, nuts, seeds, and grains while limiting or taking out creature-based nourishments. The following are a couple of tips to make the change.

• Keep it basic: pick nourishments free of added substances, additives, or engineered fixings. Even better, make everything without any preparation.

• Buy sound snacks for when you get the munchies — carrot sticks, sugar snap peas, bananas with almond spread, nuts, or a natively constructed trail blend.

• Replace natural sweetener with crude nectar, pure maple syrup, or Stevia leaf in recipes, espresso, or tea.

• Rotate new vegetables and natural products into your eating routine to keep your taste buds energized and all the more critically, to augment your supplement admission.

• Try a week after week meal prep: put aside a couple of hours out of every week to prepare nourishment in mass with the goal that you generally have perfect, solid choices close by.

• Mind your micros: certain nutrients are more earnestly to get enough of on a plant-based eating routine (e.g., iron, B-12). Include nourishments high in those supplements to your menu, or include excellent enhancements to receive every one of the rewards of plant-based eating.

A plant-based eating regimen underscores eating anything got from plants — vegetables, grains, nuts, and seeds — while limiting or barring creature determined items. While some may think a plant-based eating routine is simply another term for a vegetarian or even a vegan diet, there's an essential contrast. Plant-based eating regimens underscore eating entire, healthy nourishments and staying away from handled food sources like tofu, seitan, or bundled things — regardless of whether they're vegan or vegetarian.

Plant-Based versus Vegan and Vegetarian

Plant-based eating regimens contrast from vegan or vegetarian abstains from food in a couple of crucial ways. In the first place, let me characterize the contrast among vegans and vegetarians, however. Lacto-Ovo vegetarians take dairy and eggs, while vegans maintain a strategic distance from every creature item and typically abstain from obtaining, utilizing, and wearing items produced using or tried on creatures. Vegans and vegetarians may eat handled nourishments, similar to tofu and bundled nourishments, and may not wind up eating a sound eating regimen if such a large number of those bundled, prepared food sources end up on the menu. Individuals consuming a plant-based eating regimen, interestingly, eat entire nourishments in a structure as near nature as could be expected under the circumstances — vegetables, organic products, nuts, seeds, and so forth. Somebody following a plant-based eating routine may eat vegan or vegetarian and may pick either to utilize creature-based items or not. A few people following a by and sizeable plant-based eating routine may devour some creature items, yet it involves a little part of their eating routine.

Prepared versus Natural Food

One wellspring of perplexity is whether you can eat handled nourishment on a plant-based eating routine. Vegetarians and vegans frequently incorporate handled nourishment like locally acquired pasta, bread, wafers, or soy-based meat substitutions in their eating regimen. Those nourishments are not classified as entire food sources and in this way are not a focal piece of a plant-based eating regimen.

Instead, a plant-put together diet centers concerning getting calories from natural, entire nourishments, instead of handled ones. When eating nourishment as an whole plant-based eating regimen, you ought to likewise abstain from anything with included sugar, although you can eat things — mainly natively constructed recipes — with crude nectar, pure maple syrup, and Stevia leaf.

What Should You Eat?

Not all plant-based weight control plans are made equivalent. When following an entire nourishment plant-based eating routine, you should attempt to eat nourishments in their natural state. Cooked nourishment or food sources produced using whole grains are satisfactory — like entire grain grew bread. Continuously check the fixings list and keep away from synthetic substances, added substances, colorings, and artificial flavorings. Pick natural at whatever point conceivable. On the off chance that purchasing natural is too costly even to consider doing with each nourishment, allude to the Environmental Working Group's Dirty Dozen and Clean 15, a rundown of the most noticeably awful and best products of the soil below are some particular nourishments I suggest for a plant-based eating regimen:

Vegetables

Vegetables ought to be the establishment of any plant-based eating routine. Probably the most supplement lush plants include:
• Leafy greens: Spinach, mustard greens, kale, collard greens, Swiss chard, arugula, lettuce, micro greens (grew shoots of different sorts)
• Cruciferous vegetables: Broccoli, cauliflower, Brussels sprouts, cabbage, radishes
• Other non-dull vegetables: Eggplants, ringer peppers, avocado, okra
• Squashes: Zucchini, pumpkin, winter squash, butternut squash
• Tubers and dull greens: Sweet potatoes, parsnips, cassava, daikon, Jerusalem artichoke, ginger, beets

Organic product

Organic product, including juices, dried natural product, and crisp natural product, additionally structure a significant piece of a plant-based eating routine. You can drink organic product juice, particularly if you squeeze the natural products yourself or abstain from anything with included sugar. If you pick entire organic product over juice, you'll receive the rewards of heart-sound fibre. You can likewise eat the dried whole natural product, however, on the off chance that you are hoping to lessen your sugar admission or get more fit, limit their utilization. Although you may eat all-natural product on a plant-based eating regimen, here is a rundown of organic products with a low sugar content:

• Avocados
• Strawberries
• Grapefruit
• Raspberries
• Blueberries
• Apples
• Peaches
• Oranges
• Limes
• Olives
• Tomatoes

Vegetables
Vegetables contain heaps of macronutrients and micronutrients and are a significant wellspring of protein for plant-based eaters.

• Beans: kidney beans, lima beans, chickpeas, adzuki beans, Black beans,

• Peas: Green peas, snap peas, split peas, snow peas, dark looked at peas

• Lentils: The Red lentils, yellow lentils, green lentils, orange lentils, dark lentils

Entire Grains
All grains start complete, yet preparing strips at least one pieces of the seed orbit, just as protein from the grain. Enriched or sustained grains have had recently stripped supplements included back in — yet these are not as sound as those that held their common supplements. I suggest the accompanying entire grains (which are likewise gluten-free):

• Oats

• Millet

• Wild or darker rice

• Amaranth

• Buckwheat

• All foul flours from these entire grain sources

• Teff

• Sorghum

Fats
Some many solid fats and oils can frame a significant piece of your plant-based eating regimen. Continuously search for natural alternatives.

• Cold-squeezed oils: Avocado, sesame, additional virgin olive oil (EVOO)

• Coconut oil

Nuts and Seeds
Nuts and seeds are an extraordinary snack on a plant-based eating routine, and seeds like quinoa can be filled in as a solid grain in your meal plans.

• Seeds: Quinoa, flaxseed, hemp seeds, chia, sesame, pumpkin seeds, sunflower seeds

• Nuts: Pecans, pecans, pine nuts, Brazil nuts, cashews, cacao, hazelnuts, coconut

Nourishments to Avoid

To receive the most extreme rewards that entire, plant-inferred nourishment can give your body, psyche, and soul, take out these nourishments:

Meat

• Red meat

• Processed meat like virus cuts, bacon, lunch meat

• Seafood and shellfish

• Poultry

• Pork

Dairy and Eggs

• Milk

• Cheese

• Yoghurt

• Buttermilk

• Eggs

Prepared Foods

• Soda and caffeinated drinks

• Food with included sugar

• Refined flour

• Hydrogenated oil and trans-fats, for example, margarine.

• Refined, exceptionally handled oils with high omega-6 levels (soybean, canola, corn, cottonseed oils)

• Processed "vegan cheddar."

Plant-Based Food to Avoid

Although these are actually permitted on a plant-based eating regimen, I have found keeping away from them prompts better generally speaking wellbeing and prosperity. Point of confinement and stay away from the accompanying nourishments:

• Corn and white potatoes

• White rice

• Grains containing gluten, for example, grain, rye, wheat.

• Soybeans

• All hereditarily adjusted (GMO) nourishments

Model Plant-Based Diet Meal Plan

The accompanying meal plan is a case of what following a plant-based eating regimen could resemble.

Day One

• Breakfast: Fresh organic product beat with coconut pieces

• Lunch: Spinach plate of mixed greens with cut almonds, olives, and sun-dried tomatoes presented with a custom made a vinaigrette dressing

• Dinner: Spicy mushroom pan sear

Day Two

• Breakfast: Oatmeal with foods grown from the ground

• Lunch: Quinoa serving of mixed greens with lemon basil dressing, crisp natural product

• Dinner: Green lentil serving of mixed greens with spiced carrots, a side plate of mixed greens

Day Three

• Breakfast: Whole grain grew bread with natively constructed sunflower margarine

• Lunch: Coconut chickpea curry

• Dinner: Vegan bean stew; paprika parsnip fries with lemon cashew cream

Medical advantages of a Plant-Based Diet
Not every person pursues a plant-based eating regimen for weight loss, although that may occur if you keep eating along these lines. Individuals regularly start a plant-based eating regimen for wellbeing reasons — diminishing your danger of coronary illness, diabetes, and heftiness, for instance — or to help a progressively economical planet. The following are a portion of the advantages you may discover after receiving this inconceivable method for eating.

Get more fit
Following a plant-based eating regimen can enable you to get thinner. An oft-touted actuality is that vegetarians by and large have a lower body weight than individuals who eat both meat and vegetables. One survey of 15 investigations found that individuals who pursued a vegetarian diet on physician's instructions lost a normal of 7.5 pounds. Men who began heavier and the individuals who continued this way of eating for a more extended period lost considerably more weight. Overweight grown-ups who ate different plant-based eating regimens for a half year lost more weight than the individuals who ate meat. Vegans lost double the weight of pescatarian (individuals who eat fish yet no other meat), meat-eaters, and vegetarians. People on vegetarian weight-loss slims down additionally felt similarly full after a meal as those on meat-comprehensive diets.

Improve Your Heart Health
Plant-based weight control plans may improve your cardiovascular wellbeing by bringing down your cholesterol levels and adjusting your circulatory strain. While eats fewer carbs high in meat, dairy, and unfortunate fats may stop up arteries, vegetarian eats less, conversely, can lower blood levels of low-thickness lipoprotein (LDL or "awful" cholesterol). Individuals eating low-carb, high-protein plant-based eating regimens with sound fats may see significantly progressively articulated heart wellbeing benefits. Low-carb vegetarian diets may likewise lower glucose and blood pressure.

Lift Your Energy
A few people following a plant-based eating routine report feeling more vitality and vitality.[11] The more alarm you feel, the more you can accomplish the things you adore and the more completely you can carry on with your life. One investigation found that individuals with osteoarthritis had fundamentally more vitality, more exceptional versatility, and less everyday torment after eating a plant-based eating regimen for only two weeks contrasted and individuals eating a standard omnivorous American eating routine.

Fulfil Your Belly
The term microbiome portrays the trillions of microorganisms (microscopic organisms, growths, and infections) housed inside the gut.[13] You can develop your microbiome to have discouragement busting, corpulence battling probiotics — great organisms — by changing your eating regimen to plant-based nourishments. Matured sauerkraut, kimchi, kefir, and non-dairy yoghurt are pressed with reliable strains of intestinal microorganisms that, with standard utilization, will help build up your microbiome in a positive direction.[14] To nourish the probiotics, you need prebiotics — filaments from food sources like garlic, bananas, onions, and radishes. A plant-based eating routine can incorporate every one of these nourishments, improving your gut with each nibble.

Help Planet Earth
Eating a plant-put together diet is gentler concerning the planet. Raising animals prompts deforestation, which dispenses with natural life territory as well as intensifies environmental change by radiating ozone harming substances into the climate. Domesticated animals represent 33% of every single nursery ga outflows on the planet — more than all worldwide transportation joined — autos, trucks, trains, and planes.[15] Eating meat likewise opens people to ox-like anti-infection agents, hormones, and other pointless synthetic compounds. Diminishing meat utilization brings down asset utilization.

Supplements to Be Aware of on a Plant-Based Diet

Eating a plant-based eating regimen has such a significant number of advantages that it's difficult to trust it could do any off-base. When you maintain a strategic distance from meat and dairy, you need to ensure you get enough of specific supplements, or you could encounter insufficiencies.

Protein
As per Harvard Medical School, most vegetarians (counting individuals who pursue a plant-based eating routine) get sufficient everyday protein.[16] Many first-class competitors and Olympians have prepared and contended — and won — while buying into a solid, plant-based eating regimen. You can get the nutrients and protein your body needs from plant-based sources, including vegetables, nuts, and entire grains.

Nutrient B-12
Nutrient B-12 is discovered uniquely in creature items. If you eat a plant-based eating regimen, you could wind up with a B-12 insufficiency, except if you take an enhancement. Research demonstrates that the more significant part of vegans and 7 per cent of vegetarians are B-12 deficient. Some dairy and eggs contain B-12, Lacto-Ovo vegetarians may get enough — or may not. Certainly, all vegans and vegetarians ought to get their blood levels tried consistently and expend an exceptionally absorbable B-12 enhancement.

Iron
Since meat contains elevated levels of iron, when you stay away from it rather than plant admission, you could wind up with an iron inadequacy, which can cause sickliness. Some plant nourishments contain iron, yet you may need to search them out — alongside nourishments that lift iron retention. Phytic corrosive, a compound in some plant seeds, can keep the body from engrossing certain fundamental minerals, for example, iron, zinc, and calcium. Phytic corrosive appends to micronutrients, keeping the body from utilizing them. Taking a catalyst supplement that contains the compound phytase can help separate phytic acid.

Calcium
The vast majority who eat a plant-based eating regimen will, in general, get a lot of calcium, particularly on the off chance that they eat calcium-rich dull green verdant vegetables, similar to spinach and kale. In case you're not a fanatic of these, or you fall into a class of individuals who need a huge amount of this mineral, calcium orotate is your best decision with 90 to 95 per cent

ingestion. Calcium ought to consistently be taken with magnesium, which further guides its utilization and ingestion in the body. Nutrient D3 is likewise required for ideal calcium retention.

Omega-3 Fatty Acids (DHA)
In spite of the fact that plant-based eating regimens and omnivorous weight control plans will, in general, have equivalent admissions of α-linolenic corrosive (ALA) unsaturated fats, plant-based eating regimens will in general give less of two other omega-3 unsaturated fats: eicosapentaenoic corrosive (EPA) and docosahexaenoic corrosive (DHA) which are basic to counteracting and dealing with certain incessant conditions, including coronary heart disease. Make sure you get enough in your eating regimen.

Nutrient D
Nutrient D3 is a hormone that keeps up solid bones and equalizations calcium levels in the body, in addition to other things. And keeping in mind that our bodies produce it when presented to the bright B beams of the sun, individuals more distant from the equator are regularly nutrient D-lacking. Individuals eating a plant-based eating routine will, in general, have lower levels of D3, since this nutrient is mostly found in sustained, handled nourishment, similar to breakfast oat, juices, and margarine, or soy and bovine's milk — everything you'll evade on a plant-based diet.

Is a Plant-Based Diet Right for You?
There are limitless motivations to pursue a plant-based eating routine. First of all, you may get thinner, lessen your danger of metabolic issues and other wellbeing diseases, and you'll avoid nourishment added substances and synthetic additives. Start gradually killing dairy and meat more than a half year to one year. This steady procedure enables your body to alter and causes you to dodge reactions. These symptoms may incorporate weariness or shortcoming because of the underlying detoxification procedure of freeing the collection of meat and creature items.
Individuals taking drugs should play it safe since eating routine changes can influence how your body forms these pharmaceuticals. Plus, gradually presenting high fibre-nourishments like those in the plant-based eating regimen can help counterbalance a potential annoyed stomach that could emerge from a progressively unexpected shift. If conceivable, counsel your doctor and look for the assistance of a nutritionist before changing your eating regimen.

#FOOD BASED MISTAKES

Preparing more plant-based meals is useful for your wellbeing; for some individuals, eating more plants transform into exhausting servings of mixed greens or tasteless tofu. What's more, on the off chance that you detest what you're eating, odds are you'll go right back to the steak and chicken fingers.

Fortunately, there are a huge amount of flavors, surfaces, and hues to be found in plant-based cooking-you essentially need to move your core interest. "Cooking vegan isn't about what fixings you can't utilize; it's about the wealth of nourishments you can utilize," Open your eyes to every one of the fixings you may have disregarded previously. You can make 'frankfurter' out of farro, 'cheddar' from macadamia nuts, and 'bacon' out of shiitake mushrooms."

Eating a plant-based eating regimen is a great deal of fun. There is a different universe of vegetable love available to you when you pick plants. They are the premise of the environmental nourishment pyramid or biomass pyramid: they are the makers with the most vitality accessible. However a few followers to a plant-based way of life disregard these radiant creatures. Others fight off their craving with desserts or financially fabricated nourishment stuffs. Basically they are "low quality nourishment vegans." This doesn't need to be you, however! The following are a few hints to assist you with remaining on a way of plant-based health for a mind-blowing duration.

Here are a couple of mix-ups I see individuals make when they are beginning a plant-based way of life:

1. They don't have a care group.

We as whole need support! It tends to be hard to stay solid when you are simply beginning another method for eating. Having similarly invested individuals around you, or that you can converse with, truly makes a difference.

You could go along with one of the numerous smart dieting or gasp put together eating gatherings concerning Facebook. Take a couple of plant-based cooking classes in your locale. Pursue some plant-put together eaters concerning Instagram to get some great recipe thoughts and begin to associate with them. Join a meetup.com dinner club where you can snatch nourishment with individuals who make the most of your comparative way of life.

Nourishment is a verifiably social movement, so appreciate meeting new companions and eating and cooking together!

2. They aren't delicate with the transition.

Start gradually. Making gigantic changes before your mind has adjusted can make opposition and set you up for disappointment. Beginning gradually guarantees your prosperity, and guarantees that you are being cared to yourself, both with the transition and with giving yourself more beneficial choices.

3. They attempt to make the very same nourishments, just with plants.

Plant-based alternatives of burgers and pizza can assist you with making the transition to another method for eating and living. Yet, plant-based nourishments won't taste precisely equivalent to bacon, burgers, and cheddar stacked pizza! Plants have flavors of their own, and they are completely scrumptious.

Herbs offer alot of the flavor we've generally expected from certain global nourishments. In this way, for an Italian-roused dish, include oregano! For Indian-roused, include tumeric and cumin. Get innovative; however, on the off chance that you give it time, you will love and before long lean toward the delectable flavors of plant nourishments.

3. They eat excessively.

At the point when a few people change to plant-based, they all of a sudden start overeating themselves due to the dread of being eager. Some are even excessively worried about the protein substance of their nourishment, so they indulge and stuff themselves when they aren't ravenous, persuaded they will squander away without many grams of protein a day.

Likewise, a little yearning is a sign you are giving your body time to process and afterward detoxify. You won't bite the dust in light of the fact that your stomach is snarling for a brief period. Yearning goes back and forth and in waves. It will pass.

4. They eat pretty much nothing.

Other individuals feel solidified with their nourishment decisions, and go hungry as opposed to investigating the entire, new universe of plant-based food. They believe that everything they can eat a plate loaded with steamed broccoli and cauliflower.

I discover individuals eat too little when they are unprepared. At that point, when they feel starved, their mind dominates, and they fall directly into an undesirable, non-plant based dish. At that point, they think twice about it and begin the cycle once more!

Plant-based doesn't mean starvation. Sound plant-based eaters leave the table enjoyably fulfilled and profoundly sustained.

5. They neglect to prepare.

If there is one thing that sets individuals up to fall flat, it is neglecting to prepare.

Taking only a couple of moments to plan out your eating for the following fews days can have a significant effect. Ensure you have sound nourishments like vegetables, nuts, seeds, beans, lentils, and berries in your wash room and ice chest.

Plunge into the bright, delectable recipes that are going plant-based can offer you. Look on Instagram, read on the web. Pick recipes, make grocery lists, take as much time as is needed preparing your nourishment.

Don't feel like you need be a Michelin-featured gourmet expert. You can keep it straightforward, utilizing a couple of essential herbs and seasonings you love. Use recipes just as a rule for thoughts and flavors.

6. They attempt to enroll.

This is perhaps the greatest mix-up I see individuals make. Genuine change can happen when it originates from inside. At the point when we attempt to enroll, we are pulling somebody from their very own path of life, into our own, and it can cause hatred and enormous obstruction.

In case you're searching for help, discover it in other effectively similarly invested individuals.

7. They eat prepared vegan like Oreos and French fries.

Going plant-based is tied in with being more beneficial at the top of the priority list and body. I hear individuals constantly state that plant-based is less helpful because they are utilized to pre-bundled nourishments.

However, is that truly obvious? An apple comes prepackaged essentially.

In case you're going plant-based, be prepared. Purchase crisp fruit, vegetables, nut and seed margarine. Make straightforward, new plunges, similar to hummus. Keep a lot of little containers so you can take things in a hurry in the event that you need.

Here is a simple to pursue article about things I love to snack on when I'm in somewhat of a period crunch.

8. They are reluctant to try and stopped too early.

At the point when you weren't plant-based, you had your go-to nourishments. Truth be told, you most likely ate very similar things again and again, without contemplating it. You may stall out stuck with your plant nourishments too.

Attempt new things! Make it an objective to go out to a vegan eatery once every week, and work your way through the menu for new flavor thoughts. Research and attempt another recipe once per week, with the goal that regardless of the amount you may cherish a portion of the dishes you've made, you're attempting new things.

9. They eat heaps of starch-pasta, bread, potatoes, rice, and so on.

it is exceptionally normal.

Why? Since a great many people know about bread, pasta, rice and potatoes. They recognize how to manage them, and they are promptly accessible.

As it is, not exclusively would they be able to disrupt your weight loss endeavors, a lot of these nourishments can raise your glucose and insulin levels, and make you age quicker.

In the event that you center more around nourishments in their grungy structure (vegetables, nuts, seeds, beans, lentils, chickpeas, and so forth,), you will feel more full more and have a greatly improved possibility at getting to your ideal weight.

10. They don't make it about their wellbeing first.

Concentrating exclusively on your weight is generally insufficient to make an enduring life change.

Be that as it may, consider a portion of the advantages of a plant-based eating regimen:

- Better wellbeing, including inversion of coronary illness (world's number 1 executioner)

- Longer, more grounded life

- Lasting, increasingly sensible weight loss

- Less danger of dementia

- Increased vitality

- Environmental benefits

- No creature enduring

At the point when you become enthusiastic about your wellbeing and different ways going plant-based helps, you as well as the planet and different creatures on it, a plant-based way of life turns to be a lot simpler to support.

Indeed, the more you find out about the advantages other than simply weight loss, getting more or completely plant based gets straightforward, simple and feasible.

12. Trying too hard on the Refined Carbs

Indeed, French fries and potato chips are vegan. Would you be able to see Mr. Spock eating French fries? I don't think so. I'm grieved, he's Vulcan, however he was a plant-based eater which makes him a Vulcan vegetarian. I stray. Most bread, rice, and pasta are vegan as well, however that doesn't mean you can pig out yourself on them and still be sound! That is not legitimate. On the off chance that you have known about Dr. McDougall's The Starch Solution, you most likely feel that he advocates for a carb substantial eating regimen, regardless of the carb, yet that isn't the situation. He investigates white rice and refined grains the same amount of as other plant-based, wellbeing nourishment masters; he approves of white rice on the off chance that you eat it as a substitution for meat, frozen yogurt, and cheddar (sorry vegetarians). Fiber is your companion, and it is incredibly missing from refined carbs and your preferred seared treats. As in every way however, balance is critical. We would prefer not to see you dashing with your high fiber admission to the closest bathroom at any point in life.

13. Expending Plant-Based Fats with Gusto

Nut margarine (not nutter spreads), coconut oil, plant-based fats, goodness my! Try not to eat an entire 16 oz. sack of crude almonds since they are crude, and you believe you're eager, while viewing a film with your sibling. Try not to put coconut oil on everything in light of the fact that the bundle says it's scrumdiddlyumptious. Did you simply crush your own almond spread at the store, thinking it was cool and fun? Try not to eat the entire holder in one sitting.

14. Natural Flavors, Artificial Flavors, and Preservatives as Friends

Quit purchasing things in bundles, boxes, and packs! Nourishments contained in these kinds of bundles will in general be packed with frightful, potentially cancer-causing synthetic concoctions, that can prompt sensitivity like extreme touchiness responses and different responses. Some business nourishment added substances aren't uncovered by producers like "normal" flavors. What the hell are those? The entire world is normal from a logical viewpoint; subsequently the expression "the common world." If you couldn't care less about not recognizing what's in your nourishment, however, you can keep on putting your wellbeing in danger. What's that TV advertisement tune state? They're normally heavenly… I don't think so!

15. Seeing "Vegan" and Automatically Assuming "Solid"

Simply look at their glossy, flawless instance of vegan cupcakes and biscuits! If there are a huge number of vegan treats and items available, they are not really bravo. Numerous vegan items contain, in addition to other things, palm oil which executes orangutans while dissipated genuine sweetener is just about as "solid" as normal white sugar.

16. Purchasing Every Mock Vegan Meat Available.

Shrimp Gumbo, Shrimp Sandwich, Shrimp Stew, Shrimp Soup, all vegan, obviously. That is incredible, Bubba, however do you know precisely what's in these odd inventions? I thought not. Soy is the basic added substance in these supposed meat impostors which isn't as solid as you may might suspect. Soy has been known to make your lower lip grow and get captured out traveling wire (simply joking). No, genuinely, the primary isoflavone in soy, genistein, has been found to have hormone-upsetting properties; it impersonates estrogen, causing untimely adolescence and diminished fruitfulness, just as disturbing fetal advancement.

#OTHER WORST MISTAKES TO AVOID

Plant-based weight control plans are extremely popular, with everybody from restorative specialists to Beyoncé lauding the excellencies of a sans meat or meat-light presence. In any case, it possibly works in case you're doing it appropriately. Why miss steak in case you're committing errors?

Here are five visit slips up individuals make when beginning a plant-based diet.

1. Accepting Any Meatless Meal is Healthier

While the wellbeing science behind sourcing the majority of your nourishment from plants is sound, regardless you need to consider what you're eating: After every, french fry and lager are vegan.

Almond milk may appear to be a decent choice to dairy animals' milk, yet it just has a normal of 1.5 grams of protein per serving. What's more, numerous business brands are stacked with sugar. Essentially, white bread, pasta, potatoes and other refined carbohydrates may occupy as a lot of space in your stomach as a pork hack, yet they aren't really a shrewd decision. "Various epidemiological studies have discovered that higher admission of such carbohydrates is connected with a more serious danger of type 2 diabetes and ischemic coronary illness," composes Sharon Palmer, creator of The Plant-Powered Diet.

In case you're not eating an eating regimen offset with vegetables, fruits, entire grains, vegetables and water, you could be putting yourself in danger for weight, diabetes, coronary illness, and a large group of other wellbeing concerns. Never accept you have free rule since something is plant-based.

2. Not Getting Enough Nutrients

While it's conceivable to get every one of your nutrients and nutrients on a plant-based diet, you need to adjust your menu and way of life to ensure you consider every contingency. Nutrient B12, liable for appropriate capacity of the sensory system, is discovered basically found in creature items. A B12 inadequacy has been related with deadness, laziness, memory issues, migraines and even discouragement. Tempeh and nori have B12, and numerous vitality bars, nourishing yeasts and breakfast grains are invigorated with it, as well. Furthermore, obviously nutrient enhancements can get a move on.

Calcium consistently is by all accounts a worry with plant-based weight control plans, despite the fact that dairy animals' milk isn't the best prescribed source. The Harvard School of Public Health prescribes you, "limit milk and dairy nourishments to close to one to two servings for every day. More won't really benefit your bones in any way—and less is fine, as long as you get enough calcium from different sources."

Those "different sources" can incorporate bok choy and kale, which have higher retention rates than dairy (53% and 49%, separately, contrasted with 32% for milk). They additionally have iron and Vitamin K, which help with retaining calcium into your bones.

Omega-3 unsaturated fats, normally connected with greasy fish like salmon, lessen irritation, improve eye wellbeing, and help in bringing down the danger of coronary illness. Try not to stress, however - ocean growth, chia seeds and pecans all stockpile sufficient measures of Omega-3s.

3. Depending Too Much on Mock Meats

There's nothing amiss with tossing a veggie wiener on the flame broil or putting a tofurkey in the broiler on Thanksgiving. Meat substitutes can absolutely help with a transition to a plant-based eating routine, yet over-dependence on prepared phony meats can be counterproductive. "Many are similarly as high if not higher in fat, sodium and calories than the genuine article," dietitian Vandana Sheth disclosed to Global News. Some trendier meat choices, as Beyond Burger, have "clean marks," which just incorporate entire, characteristic or insignificantly handled fixings. In any case, many still incorporate a reiteration of fake and handled added substances to help recreate the taste and surface of meat, frequently rendering the last item very little more beneficial than the first.

In the event that despite everything you need a burger, consider patties produced using entire fixings like dark beans, sweet potatoes or quinoa. The flavor may be unique, yet it's associations superior to excessively prepared alternatives.

A similar analysis goes for artificial fromage: Many contain added substances, additives and are exceptionally prepared, some contain casein, which is a protein gotten from milk. "Cheddar" created from cashews or almonds are entire nourishments, and a sweet-potato sauce can convey a delicious macaroni and cheddar. You can likewise settle on different options all together to supplant cheddar, similar to pesto or tahini sauce.

4. Freezing Over Protein

It's an inquiry each vegan experiences: "How would you get enough protein?" To every one of those easy chair nutritionists we state: Calm down. While creature tissue has the entirety of the amino corrosive fundamental to human wellbeing does as well, rice and beans.

The day by day Recommended Dietary Allowance (RDA) for protein, is 0.36 grams per pound of body weight—that is 56 grams for the normal man, and 46 grams for a normal lady. That works out to just about 10% of your every day suggested caloric admission. Clearly in case you're dynamic or preparing for a game, you'll need more, however there are an assortment of nourishments that can supply that much protein in two or three servings. Tofu, wild rice, soy milk, oats lentils, most beans, spelt, and quinoa are your best wagers, and a few vegetables like broccoli, spinach, artichokes and brussels sprouts have around 4 to 5 grams of protein for each cooked cup.

Nourishing yeast and hemp seeds can without much of a stretch be sprinkled over a serving of mixed greens or added to a soup to pack in more protein, also.

Having one of these nourishments, and others wealthy in protein, at each meal will probably give you enough protein for the afternoon.

On the protein vein, one significant segment is expending each of the nine of the fundamental amino acids, which our bodies can't make without anyone else. Lysine is the greatest a worry in case you're vegan, since it's not very common in plant-based sources. The World Health Organization prescribes 13.6 milligrams of lysine per pound of body weight, putting the normal day by day consumption around 2,045 milligrams of lysine. Lentils and tofu are most bottomless in lysine, yet pistachios and almonds are great sources too.

5. Neglecting the Importance of Meal Planning

The vast majority currently brag a gathering of vegetarian alternatives, even at cafés. In any case, generally, deciding on a plant-based eating regimen means preparing. Remove a portion of your Sunday to prepare some plant-stuffed meals for the week is a decent method to guarantee you'll have a fair diet and not fall back on breaking your eating routine. In an example plant-based menu for tofu scramble with sauteed peppers, onions and spinach for breakfast; a burrito bowl with dark colored rice, beans, avocado, salsa and veggies for lunch; and vegetable paella with a side serving of mixed greens for dinner. Any of those can be prepared in cutting edge and heated up when you're prepared to eat.

It's a smart thought to search out new vegetarian recipes a couple of times each week, so you get variety in your eating regimen and don't fall into the snare of eating pasta, potatoes or other simple, filling meals too oftentimes. For instance, noodles made zucchini rather than refined grains offer a more beneficial option for pasta sweethearts.

In case you're going out to ear in an eatery, check the menu in advance to ensure you'll have choices. What's more, remember that some serving of mixed greens dressings and sauces may contain cream, eggs, anchovies and other creature items.

#WHAT TO BUY IN THE SUPERMARKET

Focus on the outskirts of the store. I know, you've most likely heard this previously. That is the place you'll discover the produce area, obviously, and different nourishments that are welcome in the plant-controlled eating regimen, as nondairy milks, tofu, and other soy items can be found around the edges of stores too. Some edified markets have even included mass segments for entire grains, dried vegetables, nuts, seeds, dried fruits and other such nourishments that as of not long ago must be found at the characteristic nourishments store.

Investigate the universal (or ethnic) nourishment passageway. It very well may be a decent hotspot for condiments and forte fixings that upgrade your crisp hand crafted meals. For instance, there are a wide range of sauces — teriyaki, Thai shelled nut, Indian stew sauces, that are stuffed with flavor and improve your custom made meals flawlessly. Obviously, search for brands that component common fixings and no creature items.

Solid entire nourishments are there — search for them! New fruits and vegetables, dry beans and lentils, entire grains (like darker rice and quinoa), nuts, and seeds are about as near the source as could reasonably be expected. Some insignificantly handled nourishments, still close enough to their sources, additionally have great esteem — consider nut spreads, solidified peas, natural canned beans.

Tempeh is nearer to its source (soybeans) than is tofu, however the last is likewise not an awfully prepared nourishment; both are obviously better than exceptionally handled phony meats designed from segregated soy protein. An ever increasing number of general stores are conveying nourishment and not simply "nourishment items."

Pick natural produce carefully. Truly, natural is progressively costly, however for particular sorts of produce, it's the most astute decision.

Try not to go grocery shopping when you're eager, or without a rundown close by. These are well-known inseparably tips, yet ones that bears rehashing. These propensities will in all likelihood lead to overspending and purchasing things you needn't bother with.

Peruse names cautiously. Keep away from any high fructose corn syrup item. Or then again, in case you're purchasing a prepared marinara sauce, there's no explanation behind it to have included sugar by any stretch of the imagination. In case you're going all out vegan, keep away from items that rundown gelatin, or condiments that contain fish or dairy.

On the off chance that you use coupons, ensure they're for things you truly need. Most coupons are for bundled nourishments; you'll seldom, if at any time, discover them for new produce — the nourishments we most need in our day by day charge, and which get minimal measure of promoting dollars.

Try not to succumb to marks that tout the nourishment pattern of the day. For instance, a few nourishments are normally sans gluten or low-fat. Know that bread or wafers are without gluten, however for goodness sakes, I've seen fruits and vegetables named "sans gluten." A name that expresses the reality ordinarily implies that additionally showcasing dollars are having an effect on everything.

PLANT BASED FOOD LIST TO BUY IN THE SUPERMARKET

GRAINS–

- old design oats
- rice (darker, Jasmin, wild, and so forth.)
- bulgur (a wheat grain that is extraordinary for adding surface to meatless dishes)
- quinoa
- barley (I add to soups and stews)
- millet (I add to soups and stews)
- cornmeal (for cornbread)
- grits
- unbleached flour (entire wheat, spelt, darker rice, grain, and so forth.)
- whole-wheat baked good flour
- pasta (entire wheat, spelt, artichoke, quinoa, and so forth.)
- bread (rye, pumpernickel, spelt, and so forth.)
- tortillas (corn and entire grain flour)

Vegetables Every dried and canned assortment you can consider including:

- kidney beans
- pinto beans
- garbanzo
- white beans (naval force, cannellini, incredible northern, and so forth.)
- black beans
- black-looked at peas
- green peas
- split peas
- edamame (soybean, new or solidified)
- lentils (red, green, dark colored, and so forth.)
- nuts
- many, some more…

Here's an image of my bureau and what I have close by the present moment.

VEGETABLES–

There is no restriction here. I don't keep these available. This is simply to make you mindful of what is accessible:

- potatoes (red, Russet, Yukon gold, and so on.)

- sweet potatoes
- tomatoes
- carrots
- radishes
- artichokes
- lettuces (Romaine, endive, butterhead, free leaf, and so on.)
- other greens (spinach, collards, and so on.)
- cabbages (purple, green, Napa, Bok Choy, and so on.)
- broccoli
- cauliflower
- Brussels grows
- bean grows
- leeks
- garlic
- ginger
- chime peppers (red, yellow, green)
- pepper (the hot ones)
- onions (purple, yellow, white, and so on.)
- corn
- cilantro
- parsley
- This is only a couple…

✓ FRUITS:
- apples
- pears
- oranges
- grapes
- pineapple
- nectarine
- peach
- bananas
- berries (strawberries, blueberries, raspberries, and so forth.)
- kiwi
- avocado
- lemon
- lime
- melons (melon, watermelon, honeydew, and so forth.)
- and many, some more

✓ CONDIMENTS:
- balsamic vinegar
- apple juice vinegar
- rice vinegar
- red wine vinegar
- Amino acids
- tahini (this is a sesame glue. Typically found in nutty spread segment)
- maple syrup
- blackstrap molasses
- Dijon mustard
- yellow mustard
- ketchup
- soy sauce or tamari
- Worcester sauce (ensure it doesn't have anchovies)
- vegetarian 'clam' sauce
- nutritional yeast
- sweetener, for example, sucanat or sugar (sucanat is a less refined sugar)
- baking powder
- baking pop
- corn starch or arrowroot powder (for thickening)
- vanilla
- vegan, low-fat soup cups

Flavors:

- Italian flavoring
- garlic powder
- onion powder
- paprika and smoked paprika
- peppercorn mélange
- turmeric
- tarragon
- cayenne
- chili powder
- cumin
- steak flavoring
- bay leaf
- parsley
- basil

- oregano
- red pepper pieces

CANNED FOODS:

- beans
- tomato glue
- tomato sauce
- artichoke hearts
- water chestnuts
- chipotles
- cream corn
- pimentos
- baby corn
- vegan low-fat soups
- veggie juices (Checkout article Making Veggie Stock from Scraps)
- fire-cooked tomatoes
- apple sauce

CANNED FOODS:

- hummus
- plant-based milk (soy, almond, rice, and so forth.)
- tofu (firm, additional firm, luxurious)
- tempeh
- seitan
- lemon juice
- flax meal
- salsa

FROZEN FOODS:

- Ezekiel bread (they are kept in the cooler area of numerous grocery stores)
- hash tans
- fruits (like berries, and so forth.)
- chopped spinach
- corn snack
- green peas

- mixed veggies
- stir fry veggies
- healthy plant-based pizza outside layers
- whole-grain bagels
- whole-grain buns (for bean burgers and carrot franks)

#A PLANT-BASED SHOPPING LIST FOR A LEAN AND STRONG BODY and MIND

The most ideal approach to show this appeared to be to separated the nourishments I purchase in mass (normally a month to month premise) versus the food sources I purchase week by week (generally crisp produce). I've additionally gone above and beyond and gave an 'on a spending plant-based/vegan grocery list'.

1. Legumes: 3 serves for each day (this can be beans, lentils, chickpeas, natural plunges like bean plunge/hummus or softly handled vegetable items like tofu and tempeh)

2. Whole Grains: 3+ serves every day (dark colored rice, oats, entire wheat pasta, quinoa, wild rice, buckwheat are my gauges)

3. Dark Leafy Greens: 2-3 servings for each day

4. Cruciferous Vegetables (broccoli, broccolini, cauliflower, and so on): 1 serve for each day

5. Other Vegetables: 3+ serves every day (sweet potato and carrots are two of my top picks)

6. Berries: 2-3 serves day. (Berries are low calorie thus high in hostile to disease and cardiovascular defensive phytonutrients/cancer prevention agents that I believe it's basic you get 2-3 serves in a day)

7. Other Fruits: 3 serves for every day (e.g., banana, kiwi fruit, and pears)

8. Omega 3 Seeds: 1-2 serves for every day (hemp seeds, flax meal, chia seeds)

9. Nuts: 1-3 serve for every day (pecans, brazil nuts, almonds are my best 3)

10. Fermented Foods: sauerkraut, kimchi, miso Soup, kefir.

11. Spices: 1 serve for every day (turmeric and ground ginger a day are my top picks).

COMMON PLANT BASED DIET SUPPLEMENT

•Cyanocobalamin and have composed a blog on this here

•   Vitamin D: If you are not ready to get 20 mins of sun a day with your hands and face uncovered. I suggest a 1000-2,000 IU supplement. Ensure it's sourced from Vitamin D2 (plant structure) or if it's from Vitamin D3 it unmistakably says its sourced from Lichen. All other Vitamin D3 is sourced from creatures.

•   Omega 3 DHA Algae Oil: If you are not expending a couple of serves of hemp, chia or flax seeds every day. Keep in mind, on an entire directly long chain Omega 3's shows improvement over somebody on a creature based eating regimen so in the event that you are having adequate hemp, chia as well as flaxseed meal in your eating regimen then you needn't bother with this enhancement.

Different enhancements are best guided by a blood test and decided in meeting with a Dietician, Nutritionist or potentially Doctor.

In the event that you adhere to the suggested serves per gathering/day and take your Vitamin B 12 (and conceivable Vitamin D/Omega 3 Algae oil) you will arrive at all the nutrient necessities that your body needs to totally flourish and you will be free from cholesterol, immersed creature fats, creature protein, anti-microbials and hormones that unleash ruin in your body and have been appeared to build your odds of creating incessant illness. I suggest running your eyes over the Plant Proof Healthy Vegan Food Pyramid I as of late made and in any event, printing a duplicate to have in your kitchen until you feel certain with this better approach for consuming.

THE NATURE OF FOODS TO BE KEPT IN THE FREEZER

I separated them into nourishments I purchase in BULK and generally most recent multi month or more and food sources I purchase crisp week by week.

Mass FOODS:

1.   The Hemp seeds, ground flaxseed and (we don't process entire flaxseeds. Best wager is to get them entire and granulate what you need crisp each Chia Seeds time you expend them)

2.   Hemp as well as Pea Protein Powder (not to supplant entire nourishments, just as an enhancement for somebody who is too dynamic and is as of now eating the recommended number of entire food sources a day).

3.   Oats or potentially Lupin Flakes (natural Lupin just prescribed because of herbicides utilized in non-regular Lupin cultivating)

4.   Nuts (Almonds, Walnuts, Brazil Nuts, Pine Nuts as a rule)

5.   Quinoa

6.   Brown and Wild Rice

7.   Legumes (Beans, Chickpeas and Lentils). Spots like Woolworths sell natural canned beans for $1.50 or under. Likewise, exceptionally suggest getting crude beans and drenching for a couple of meals seven days. Likewise an extraordinary method to fuse beans into your eating routine on the off chance that you discover them hard on your stomach (gas/swelling). Peruse progressively about how to battle gas, swelling and tooting on a plant based or vegan diet here.

8.   Fresh Basil, Coriander, Parsley, Mint, Chives

9.   Extra-Virgin Olive Oil (to utilize sparingly whenever required)

10.   Nutritional Yeast

New FOODS:

1.   Tempeh (Organic Village Chickpea Tempeh and Organic Village dark bean Tempeh yet a Non-GMO soy tempeh is added to fine in the event that you can't get Organic Villlage Tempeh or comparative in your general vicinity).

2.   Avocado

3.   Organic Non-GMO Tofu

4.   Dark Leafy Greens (Kale, Collards, the Custard Greens and Spinach)

5.   Cruciferous Vegetables (, Cabbage, Brussel Sprouts, Broccoli, Cauliflower, Bok Choy Broccolini).

6.   Other Vegetebales (Mushrooms, Cucumber, Zucchini, Fresh Beetroot)

7.   Sauerkraut

8.   Berries (Blueberries, Blackberries, Strawberries)

9.   Other Fruits (Banana, Pineapple, Apricots)

10.   Nut Milk (Soy, Hazelnut, Almond, , Macadamia and Cashew commonly)

11.   Turmeric, Mustard Seed Powder, Pink Sea Salt Cayenne Pepper, Cumin, , Cracked Pepper, Wakame Flakes

12.   Coconut and Organic Soy Yogurt (go for one that is low sugar and just contains the common fats)

13.   Cocoa Nibs or Cacao Powder

AN ATHLETE, A PREGNANT WOMAN AND A PERSON DESIRING TO LOSE WEIGHT PLAJNT DIET MEAL SHOPPING LIST

These are the nourishments and nutrition classes that I suggest for everybody. Your objectives and individual conditions will at that point manage what measure of nourishment you buy, what meals you prep and how as often as possible you eat. For instance, pregnant ladies might need to concentrate more on vegetables that offer folate and iron like beetroot.

Inside the prescribed nourishment classifications, you can obviously stay away from specific food sources in the event that you have explicit dietary contemplations (e.g celiac).

Outline OF MY PLANT-BASED OR VEGAN GROCERY SHOPPING LIST TIPS:

The incredible thing about the above is that most of the nourishments are open to everybody and are far less expensive than purchasing meat, fish, and so on. On the off chance that you search for BULK supply stores close by, you can spare every day by loading up on the 'Mass nourishments list' ahead of time (less expensive per KG). On the off chance that the 11 nourishment classifications appear to be a bit of overpowering, simply consider your standard meals. Numerous meals contain nourishments that range over a few of these classes so you will tick them off simultaneously.

Thinking about whether you ought to purchase natural or customary produce? You can peruse my particular blog on this point however to put it plainly, indeed, natural produce will restrict your introduction to terrible pesticides/herbicides like glyphosate (gather together) which has been connected to an expanded possibility of creating disease. In the event that financial limit is an issue, at that point eating ordinary produce is still surely superior to keeping away from fruit and vegetables when all is said in done as they contain such a large number of nutrients to pass up. In my blog on natural versus regular produce, I have made a table that shows the best 10 nourishments to purchase as natural where conceivable as these normally contain the most pesticides/herbicides (e.g strawberries).

At the point when you start eating this way, it's normal for your body to set aside some effort to change. Much the same as in the event that you move from an excessively chilly area to a steaming hot and muggy area – the human body sets aside some effort to settle. Above your first month transitioning to a plant-based diet, your gut microorganisms (which as of not long ago probably contains microscopic organisms dependent on eating a great deal of meat and negligible vegetables and probiotic nourishments) will start to experience their very own change. This is an extremely positive procedure, as the decent variety of your sound microscopic organisms will increment quickly, so on the off chance that you see some stomach thunders or possibly a minor piece of swelling, simply recollect this is absolutely ordinary and you are acquainting your body with something totally new. Over the long haul once your framework has grown new gut microbes you won't think back and will be really blossoming with clean entire nourishment plant-based sustenance.

RECIPES

1. BREAKFAST RECIPES

BREAKFAST RECIPES

VANILLA CHIA PUDDING

Makes 2 Servings

Fixings

6 tablespoons chia seeds

2 cups almond milk

2 tablespoon maple syrup or agave

1 teaspoon vanilla concentrate

1/2 teaspoon cinnamon

Technique

1. Mix the almond milk, vanilla, maple syrup, and cinnamon.

2. Pour fluid blend over the chia seeds and mix till seeds are equally blended in. Mix again five minutes after the fact, and five minutes after that. Let sit for an hour in any event, or just let it sit in the refrigerator medium-term. Serve, bested with a crisp product of decision. Pudding will keep in the fridge for as long as four days.

QUINOA BREAKFAST PORRIDGE

Serves 2-4

Fixings

1 cup dry quinoa

2 cups almond milk

1 tbsp agave or maple syrup

1/2 tsp vanilla

1/2 tsp cinnamon

1 tablespoon ground flax meal

Discretionary toppers and include ins: cut banana, new berries, a couple of tablespoons crude pecans, 1 tablespoon of chia seeds, 1 tablespoonful of almond margarine

Technique

1. Combine quinoa, almond milk, sugar, vanilla, and cinnamon in a little pot. Warm to the point of boiling and lessen to a stew.

2. Allow the quinoa to cook until the majority of the fluid is retained, and quinoa is fleecy (15-20 minutes). Blend in the flax meal. Blend in any extra toppers or include ins, and appreciate.

Scraps will keep in the ice chest for as long as three days and can be warmed with almond milk over the stove.

BANANA AND ALMOND BUTTER OATS

Serves 2

Fixings

1 cup gluten-free moved oats

1 cup almond milk

1 cup of water

1 teaspoon cinnamon

2 tablespoons almond spread

1 banana, cut

Strategy

1. Mix the water and almond milk to a bubble in a little pot. Add the oats and diminish to a stew.

2. Cook until oats have consumed all fluid. Blend in cinnamon. Top with almond spread and banana and serve.

GLUTEN-FREE, VEGAN BANANA PANCAKES

Serves 2-3

Fixings

1 cup generally useful, gluten-free flour

1/2 tsp preparing powder

1/2 tsp cinnamon dash ocean salt

1 tsp apple juice vinegar

2/3 cup almond milk

1 ready banana

1 teaspoon vanilla

1 tbsp + 2 tsp dissolved coconut oil, isolated

Strategy

1. Mix the flour, preparing powder, cinnamon, and ocean salt together.
2. Mix the vinegar to the almond milk and whisk together till foam. Include the almond/vinegar blend to a blender, alongside the banana, vanilla, and 1 tbsp coconut oil. Mix till smooth.
3. Mix the fluid blend into the flour blend till consolidated.

4. Warm 2 tsp coconut oil in a nonstick skillet. Include the hitter, storing 1/4 cup at once. Give the hotcakes a chance to cook till air pockets structure on the top; at that point, flip and keep cooking till flapjacks are cooked through. Rehash with all outstanding hitter.

5. Serve flapjacks with new berries.

APPLE CINNAMON OATMEAL

Serves 2

Fixings

1 cup gluten-free moved oats

1 cup of water

3/4 cup almond milk

3/4 cup diced apples

1/2 teaspoon cinnamon or pumpkin pie zest

2 tbsp maple syrup

1/4 cup slashed crude pecan pieces

Technique

1. Combine the oats, water, almond milk, apples, cinnamon, and syrup in a medium pot or pan. Heat to the point of boiling and lower to a stew. Cook until oats have assimilated. The fluid and apples are delicate (around 10-15 minutes).

2. Divide oats into two dishes and top with crude pecan pieces. Appreciate.

STRAWBERRY GINGER CHIA PUDDING

Makes 2 servings

Fixings

6 tbsp chia seeds

1 cup solidified or healthy strawberries

1 3/4 cups almond milk

3/4 tsp ginger powder (substitute cinnamon if you like)

1 tablespoon maple syrup

Strategy

1. Mix the strawberries, milk, ginger, and sugar on high till smooth.

2. Pour fluid over the chia seeds and mix each couple of minutes for the following fifteen minutes.

BANANA BREAKFAST WRAPS

Serves 2

Fixings

2 enormous bananas

4 Boston or margarine lettuce leaves

4 tbsp almond margarine

4 tsp maple syrup

Technique

1. Spread every lettuce leaf with a tablespoon of almond margarine.

2. Cut the bananas down the middle. Spot half of a banana in each leaf. Sprinkle each with a teaspoon of maple syrup and serve.

GLUTEN-FREE, VEGAN PUMPKIN MUFFINS

Makes 12 biscuits

Fixings

2 cups gluten-free, generally useful flour

2 tsp preparing powder

1 tsp heating pop

2 tsp pumpkin pie zest

1/2 tsp. salt

1 teaspoon apple juice vinegar

1 cup almond milk

2 tbsp softened coconut oil

1/2 cup maple syrup

3/4 cup pumpkin puree

1/2 cup raisins (discretionary)

Technique

1. Preheat grill to 350 degrees daintily oils a biscuit tin.

2. Mix the flour, heating powder, preparing pop, pumpkin pie flavor, and salt in a considerable blending bowl.

3. In a different blending bowl, whisk together the apple juice vinegar and almond milk till foamy. Blend in the oil, syrup, and pumpkin puree.

4. Pour the wet fixings into the dry fixings and blend till they're joined—don't overmix — overlay in the raisins.

5. Spoon the player into biscuit tins and prepare for around 20-25 minutes, or until a toothpick embedded into the major part of a biscuit tells the truth. Cookies will keep for as long as three days in a sealed shut holder or can be solidified.

2. LUNCH RECIPES

RED CABBAGE AND GREEN APPLE SESAME SLAW

Serves 2

Fixings

For the plate of mixed greens:

3 cups daintily destroyed red cabbage

1 huge granny smith apple, destroyed

2 tbsp hemp seeds

For the dressing:

1/4 cup tahini

3 tablespoons water

2 teaspoons agave nectar or maple syrup

1/2 teaspoon sesame oil

1/2 – 1 tsp ocean salt (to taste)

1 tablespoon apple juice vinegar

Technique

1. Whisk dressing fixings together and put in a safe spot.

2. Dress the destroyed vegetables and hemp seeds with dressing; you can use as much as you can imagine, however, ensure you coat everything great (a half-cup will likely get the job done). Serve. Slaw will keep in the ice chest medium-term.

Serves 2

Fixings

For the serving of mixed greens:

5 cups washed, dried, and slashed kale (around 1 bundle after preparation)

2 little carrots, ground

2 stalk celery, slashed

4 tbsp brilliant raisins

4 tbsp slashed pecans

1 apple, cut meager

For the dressing:

2 tbsp olive oil

1/2 tbsp apple juice

1 tbsp agave

Salt and pepper to taste

Technique

1. Whisk the dressing fixings together, and put in a safe spot.

2. In a significant blending bowl, pour about the dressing onto the slashed kale and start "rubbing" it with your hands until the kale begins to get delicate and all around covered. It ought to grow even a withered surface.

2. Add the rest of the plate of mixed greens fixings, and prepare the entire serving of mixed greens once more.

3. Plate the serving of mixed greens, and top it with your cut apple. Appreciate. Remains will keep medium-term in the refrigerator.

SMOKY AVOCADO AND JICAMA SALAD

Serves 2

Fixings

For the dressing:

One little avocado

1 tbsp cumin powder

Juice of 2 limes

1/2 teaspoon smoked paprika

1 cup of water

1/4 tsp salt

Run cayenne pepper

For the plate of mixed greens:

1 piling cup destroyed cabbage

1 piling cup destroyed carrot

10 huge leaves romaine lettuce, cut meagerly

2 cups jicama, cut into matchsticks

2 tbsp toasted pumpkin seeds

Strategy

1. Blend all dressing fixings in a blender or processor till smooth.

2. Pour dressing over this plate of mixed greens, and hurl. Serve.

MANGO, KALE, AND AVOCADO SALAD

Serves 2

Fixings:

1 pack wavy kale, de-stemmed, slashed, washed, and dried (around 6 cups after preparation)

Juice of 1 enormous lemon

2 teaspoons flax or olive oil

1 teaspoon sesame oil

2 teaspoons maple syrup or agave nectar

Ocean salt to taste.

1 hacked red ringer pepper

1 cup mango, cut into little 3D squares

1 little Haas avocado, cut into 3D squares

Strategy

1. "Massage" the lemon juice, flax/olive and sesame oils, syrup, and salt into the kale till it's dried and dressed equitably.

2. Mix in the pepper, mango, and avocado 3D squares. Hurl well to join. Serve.

SIMMERED BUTTERNUT SQUASH AND APPLE SOUP

Makes 4 servings

Fixings

1 butternut squash, stripped and hacked (around 3-4 lbs, or 4-5 cups)

3 little apples, generally hacked

1 little onion, hacked

2 tbsp dissolved coconut oil

1/2 tsp legitimate or ocean salt (+more to taste)

Dark pepper to taste

1/4 tsp nutmeg

1/2 tsp squashed thyme

2 1/2 cups low sodium vegetable soup

1/2 cup canned coconut milk

Strategy

1. Place squash, apples, and onion on a huge simmering plate. Sprinkle coconut oil and salt and pepper over them, blend with your hands, and dish at 376 degrees for around 45 minutes, or until they're all delicate and brilliant.

2. Place broiled veggies in a blender with vegetable stock, nutmeg, coconut milk, and thyme. If the soup needs progressively fluid, include some more, until it arrives at the consistency you like.

3. Transfer soup to a pot, re-warmth, and serve.

SIMPLE CURRIED YELLOW LENTILS WITH AVOCADO "Bread garnishes."

Serves 4

Fixings

3/4 cup onion, diced

1/2 tbsp coconut oil

1 cup yellow lentils

1 bowl of sweet potato, cut into 1/2 inch 3D shapes

2 carrots, diced (discretionary, yet I had them, so I utilized them!)

1/2 tsp turmeric

1 tbsp gentle curry powder

1 tsp powdered ginger

1/2 tsp ocean salt

Dark pepper to taste

4 cups vegetable soup or water

Strategy

1. Heat oil in a massive pot over medium warmth. Saute onion till its turning translucent and somewhat brilliant. Include the lentils, potato, carrots, and flavours/seasonings, and blend to consolidate everything.

2. Add the juices or water to the pot and heat to the point of boiling. Diminish to a stew and cook for 25 minutes, or until the lentils and sweet potato are delicate.

3. Allow lentils to cool somewhat, at that point present with new avocado cuts.

KALE SALAD WITH CARROTS, APPLES, RAISINS, AND CREAMY CURRY DRESSING

Serves 2-4

Fixings

For the dressing:

1/2 cup crude cashews or pecans

2 tablespoons lemon juice

2 set dates

1/2 cup water

1/2 tsp ocean salt

2 tsp curry powder

For the plate of mixed greens:

1 head kale, de-stemmed, washed, dried, and cut into scaled-down pieces (around 5 cups)

2 huge carrots, stripped and hacked

1 huge apple, hacked into little pieces

1/3 cup raisins

1/2 cup chickpeas

Strategy

1. Blend all dressing fixings in a rapid blender till smooth.

2. Massage the kale with the dressing, ensuring that everything is all around covered and mellowed (start with 1/2 cup dressing and include as required—you may have some remaining). Include the apple, carrot, raisins, and chickpeas, and remix the serving of mixed greens, including all the more dressing on the off chance that you like. Serve.

RED QUINOA, ALMOND AND ARUGULA SALAD WITH CANTALOUPE

Makes 2 servings

Fixings

1/2 cups crisp melon, cut into 1-inch pieces

1/2 cups red quinoa (customary quinoa is additionally absolutely beautiful)

4 cups arugula, firmly pressed

1/4 cup fragmented, disintegrated, or cut almonds

2 tablespoons flax, hemp, or olive oil

1 tablespoon apple juice vinegar

2
1 teaspoon maple syrup

Ocean salt and dark pepper to taste

Strategy

1. Whisk together the oil, vinegar, syrup, and flavouring.

2. Divide the arugula, quinoa, and melon onto two serving plates. Sprinkle them with almonds and afterwards shower the dressing over them.

HOT THAI SALAD

Serves 2

Fixings

For the dressing:

1 avocado

1 cup of coconut water

¼ cup cilantro

¼ cup basil

¼ tsp salt (or progressively) 2 set dates

1 tbsp minced or ground ginger Sprinkle of cayenne pepper

For the plate of mixed greens:

1 chime pepper, slashed

2 cups ground carrots

1/2 cup cilantro, hacked

1 cup grows

2 cups destroyed romaine lettuce

1 cup cut cucumbers
Strategy

1. Blend all dressing fixings in a rapid blender till smooth.

2. The top plate of mixed greens with dressing as wanted. Serve.

CARROT AVOCADO BISQUE

Serves 2

Fixings

2 cups carrot juice

1/2 Haas avocado

1 tablespoon low sodium tamari

1 teaspoon ground ginger

Strategy

Mix all fixings in a rapid blender till smooth.

GLUTEN-FREE TORTILLA PIZZA

Serves 2

Fixings

2 10" darker rice tortillas (Food for Life brand)

2/3 cup low sodium, natural marinara sauce, isolated

2 cups vegetable + garnishes of decision (broccoli, spinach, peppers, mushrooms, olives, artichokes, cooked potato, and so on)

1/2 cup fundamental cashew cheddar (formula beneath)

Technique

1. Preheat grill to 400 F. Spot tortillas on a foil or material lined heating sheet. Prepare for 5-

8 minutes, or until marginally fresh.

2. Remove tortillas from broiler. Top with tomato sauce and veggies, and come back to the grill for 8-

10 more minutes (till garnishes are cooked through). Speck with cashew cheddar, and serve.

NB: If you don't have cashew cheddar, you can sprinkle pizzas with nourishing yeast.

You can likewise utilize red pepper hummus instead of the tomato sauce.

CASHEW CHEESE

Makes 1 cup

Fixings

1/4 cups cashews, splashed for in any event three hours (or medium-term) and depleted 1/2 tsp ocean salt

1 little clove garlic, minced (discretionary)

2 tbsp lemon juice

1/3-1/2 cup water

1/4 cup nourishing yeast

Technique

Spot the cashews, ocean salt, garlic, lemon, and 1/3 cup water in a nourishment processor. Procedure till the blend is exceptionally smooth and delicate (you're going for a surface like velvety ricotta cheddar), halting to scratch the bowl down a couple of times and including some additional water as vital.

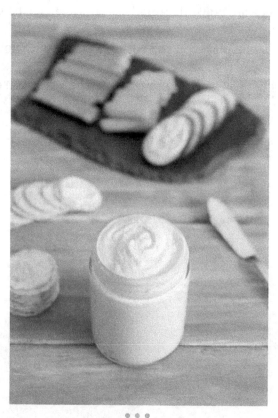

COOKED CAULIFLOWER AND PARSNIP SOUP

Yields 4 servings

Fixings

1 medium head cauliflower, cleaved

4 huge parsnips, stripped and slashed

1-2 tbsp olive oil

4 shallots, cut down the middle

1 clove garlic, minced

1 tsp thyme

1/2 tsp sage

4 cups vegetable stock

1/2 cup almond or coconut milk

Ocean salt and pepper to taste

Paprika

Strategy

1. Preheat stove to 400 degrees. Line a preparing plate or two with tin foil.

2. Lay cauliflower, parsnips, shallots, and garlic, out on foil, and shower with olive oil, thyme, wine, salt and pepper.

3. Roast veggies for around 35-40 min, or until they're delicate and brilliant dark coloured.

4. Place veggies in a rapid blender (you may need to work in groups) and include stock and non-dairy milk. Mix until soup is smooth and creamy, including progressively fluid on the off chance that you have to. On the other hand, you can utilize an inundation blender.

5. Transfer soup to a pot and re-season to taste with salt and pepper.

3. DINNER RECIPES

DARK BEAN AND QUINOA SALAD WITH QUICK CUMIN DRESSING

Serves 4

Fixings

For the serving of mixed greens:

1 cup dry quinoa, flushed

Run salt

2 cups vegetable juices or water

1/2 enormous cucumber, diced flawlessly

1 little ringer pepper, diced flawlessly

1 can BPA free, natural dark beans

10-15 basil leaves, hacked into a chiffonade

1/4 cup new cilantro, hacked

For the vinaigrette:

2 tbsp additional virgin olive oil

1/4 cup apple juice vinegar

1 tbsp agave or maple syrup

1 tbsp dijon mustard

1 tsp cumin

Salt and pepper to taste

Strategy

1. Rinse quinoa through a strainer till the water runs clear. Move it to a little or medium estimated pot and include two cups of vegetable juices or water and run of salt. Spread the bowl with the

goal that the top is on, yet there's a little hole where water can getaway. Stew till quinoa has ingested the majority of the fluid and is feathery (around 15-20 minutes).

2. Transfer cooked quinoa to a blending bowl. Include cleaved vegetables, dark beans, and herbs.

3. Whisk dressing fixings. Add the dressing to the plate of mixed greens, and serve.

1) Serving of mixed greens will keep for three days in the ice chest.

ZUCCHINI PASTA WITH, BASIL, SWEET POTATO, HEMP PARMESAN AND CHERRY TOMATOES

Serves 2

Fixings

2 enormous zucchini

1 red ringer pepper, diced

15 cherry tomatoes, quartered

8 enormous basil leaves, chiffonaded

2 little sweet potato, heated and after that cut into solid shapes

2 tbsp balsamic vinegar

1 little avocado, cubed

4 tbsp hemp parmesan (formula beneath)

Technique

1. Use the spiralizer to cut zucchini into long strips (looking like noodles).

2. Toss zucchini with every single residual fixing, and serve.

Hemp Parmesan

Makes 1/2 - 2/3 cup

Fixings

6 tbsp hemp seeds

6 tbsp nourishing yeast

Run ocean salt

Technique

Join all fixings in a nourishment processor, and heartbeat to separate and consolidate. Store in the refrigerator for as long as about fourteen days.

GLUTEN-FREE WHITE BEAN AND SUMMER VEGETABLE PASTA

Serves 4

Fixings

1 little eggplant, cut into 1-inch 3D squares and gently salted for 30 minutes, at that point tap dry

1 clove garlic, minced

1 would organically be able to fire simmered, diced tomatoes

1 little can natural tomato sauce

1 tsp agave

1 tbsp dried basil

1 tsp dried oregano

1 tsp dried thyme

1 can (or 2 cups newly cooked) cannellini or naval force beans, depleted

8 oz. dry dark coloured rice or quinoa pasta (rigatoni, linguine, and penne are on the whole fine)

Strategy

1. Heat a considerable skillet with olive or coconut oil shower (or utilize a couple of tbsp water).

2. Add the zucchini and cook it till delicate.

3. Include the canned tomatoes, agave, basil, oregano, tomato sauce, thyme. Warmth through. Test for flavouring, and include a higher amount of whatever herbs you like.

4. Add the white beans and warmth the entire sauce through. This is so delectable and basic, and you could eat it all alone as a "cheaters.

5. When your sauce is cooking, put a pot of salted water to bubble. Include pasta when it hits a moving bubble, and cook pasta till delicate yet at the same time somewhat still somewhat firm.

6. Drain pasta, cover with sauce and serve.

Remains will keep for three days in the cooler.

BUTTERNUT SQUASH CURRY

Serves 4

Fixings

1 tablespoon dissolved coconut oil

1 white or yellow onion, hacked

1 clove garlic, minced

1 tablespoon new ginger, minced

3 tablespoons red curry glue

1 tablespoon natural sugar or coconut sugar

2/3 cups vegetable soup

One 14-or 15-ounce would coconut be able to drain.

One green or red ringer pepper, hacked.

2-pound butternut squash

1 cups green beans, cut into 2" pieces

1 to 2 tablespoon lime juice

Technique

1. Heat the coconut oil in an enormous pot or wok. Include the onion and cook till it's delicate and translucent (5 to 8 minutes).

2. Mix the garlic and ginger, let them cook for about a moment. At that point, include the curry glue and sugar. Combine the fixings until the glue is equitably fused.

3. Whisk in the juices, the coconut milk, and the tamari. Include the red pepper and butternut squash. Stew till the squash is delicate (25 to 30 minutes). If you have to include additional stock as the blend cooks, do as such.

4. Mix the green beans and let them cook for a few minutes, or until delicate. Season the curry to taste with additional soy sauce or tamari and mix in the lime squeeze as wanted. Expel from warmth and serve over quinoa or dark coloured basmati rice.

Remains will keep for four days.

CRUDE ZUCCHINI ALFREDO WITH BASIL AND CHERRY TOMATOES

Serves 2 (with remaining alfredo sauce)

Fixings

Pasta

Two huge zucchini

1 cup cherry tomatoes, split

1/4 cup basil, cut

Crude alfredo sauce

1 cup cashews, splashed for in any event three hours (or medium-term) and depleted 1/3 cup water

1 tsp agave or maple syrup

1 clove garlic

3-4 tbsp lemon juice (to taste)

1/4 cup dietary yeast

1/4 tsp ocean salt

1. Use a spiralizer and cut the zucchini into different long strips.

2. Add the tomatoes and basil to the zucchini noodles and put them regardless of in a huge blending bowl.

3. Blend the majority of the alfredo sauce fixings in a rapid grinder till smooth.

4. Cover the pasta in 1/2 cup sauce, and blend it in well, including extra sauce as required

(you'll have some sauce extra). Serve.

DARK BEAN AND CORN BURGERS

Makes 4 Burgers

Fixings

1 tablespoon coconut oil

1 little yellow onion, cleaved

1 cup new, solidified or canned natural corn bits

1 can natural, low sodium dark beans, depleted (or 1/2 cups cooked dark beans)

1 cup dark coloured rice, cooked

1/4 cup oat flour (or ground, moved oats)

1/4 cup tomato glue

2 tsp cumin

One loading tsp paprika

1 loading tsp bean stew powder

1/2 - 1 tsp ocean salt (to taste)

Dark pepper or red pepper, to taste

Technique

1. Preheat your broiler to 350 F.

2. Heat the coconut oil in an enormous sauté container. Include the onion and saute till onion is brilliant, delicate, and fragrant (around 5-8 minutes).

2) Add corn, beans, and tomato glue to the container and warmth through.

3) Place the cooked rice into the bowl of a nourishment processor. Include the beans, onion, tomato glue, and corn blend. Heartbeat to join. Include flavours, oat flour, and a bit of water if you need it. Pulse more, until you have a thick and clingy (yet malleable) blend. If the mixture is excessively wet, include a tablespoon or two of extra oat flour.

4) Shape into 4 burgers and spot burgers on a foil-lined heating sheet. Heat for 25 - 30 minutes, or until burgers are delicately crisped, flipping once through. Present with new guacamole, whenever wanted!

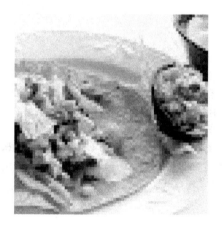

EGGPLANT ROLLATINI WITH CASHEW CHEESE

Serves 4

Fixings

For rollatini:

2 huge eggplant, cut the long way into 1/4 inch thick cuts Olive oil

1/4 cups cashews, splashed for in any event three hours (or medium-term) and depleted 1/2 tsp ocean salt

1 little clove garlic, minced (discretionary)

2 tbsp lemon juice

1/3-1/2 cup water

1/4 cup dietary yeast

2 tsp dried basil

1 tsp dried oregano

Dark pepper to taste

1/2 10 oz. bundle solidified spinach, defrosted and crushed altogether to evacuate all overabundance fluid (I press mine immovably through a strainer)

1/2 cups natural, low sodium marinara sauce

Technique

1. Preheat grill to 400 F. Cut eggplants the long way into strips around 1/2" thick. Spot eggplant cuts onto preparing sheets and sprinkle well with ocean salt or fit salt. Let sit for

30 minutes; this declines sharpness and evacuates abundance dampness. Pat the cuts dry, and shower them or brush them daintily with olive oil.

2. Roast eggplant cuts till searing (around 20 min), flipping part of the way through.

3. While eggplant is broiling, make the cashew cheddar. Spot the cashews, ocean salt, garlic, lemon, and 1/3 cup water in a nourishment processor. Procedure till the blend is exceptionally smooth and delicate (you're going for a surface like velvety ricotta cheddar), halting to scratch the

bowl down a couple of times and including some additional water as fundamental. Stop the engine, and include the fresh yeast, basil, oregano, and dark pepper. Procedure again to consolidate. Move the cashew cheddar to a bowl and blend in the slashed spinach. Put the cheddar blend in a safe spot.

4. Remove the cooked eggplant from the grill and lessen warmth to 325 F. Enable the cuts to cool until they can be taken care of. Move them to a cutting board and include around 3 tbsp of the cheddar blend as far as possible of one side. Move up from that side, and spot crease down in a little meal dish. Rehash with every single residual cut.

5. Smother the eggplant moves with tomato sauce, and heat, revealed, for around 20-25 minutes, or until hot. Present with sides of the decision.

GINGER LIME CHICKPEA SWEET POTATO BURGERS

Makes 4-6 Burgers

Fixings

3/4 cup cooked chickpeas

1/2 little onion

1-inch ginger slashed

1 tsp coconut oil

1/2 cups sweet potato, heated or steamed and cubed 1/3 cup quinoa drops or gluten-free moved oats

Two piling tbsp flax meal

2-3 tbsp lime juice (to taste)

2 tbsp low sodium tamari

1/4 cup cilantro, hacked

Run red pepper chips (discretionary)

Water as required

Strategy

1. Preheat stove to 350 F.

2. Heat coconut oil in a large dish or wok. Saute onion 2 tsp coconut oil (or coconut oil shower) till delicate and fragrant (around 5 minutes). Include chickpeas and warmth through.

3. Place the chickpeas, ginger, and onion in a nourishment processor and include the sweet potato, quinoa drops or oats, flaxseed, lime juice, cilantro, tamari or coconut aminos, and run of red pepper pieces, if utilizing. Heartbeat to join, at that point, run the engine and include some water until the consistency is thick yet straightforward to form.

4. Shape blend into 4-6 burgers. Heat at 350 degrees for around 35 minutes, flipping partially through.

SWEET POTATO AND BLACK BEAN CHILI

Serves 6

Fixings

1/2 cup dried dark beans.

5 cups sweet potato, diced into 3/4 inch shapes

One tablespoon olive oil

1/2 cups slashed white or yellow onion

Two cloves garlic, minced

1 chipotle pepper en adobo, slashed finely

2 teaspoons cumin powder

1/2 teaspoon smoked paprika

1 tablespoon ground bean stew powder

1 14 or 15-ounce jar of natural, diced tomatoes (I like the Muir Glen brand)

1 can natural, low sodium dark beans (or 1/2 cups cooked dark beans)

2 cups low sodium vegetable soup, Sea salt to taste

Strategy

1. Warm the tablespoon of oil in a dutch stove or an enormous pot. Saute the onion for sometimes, at that point include the sweet potato and garlic. Keep sauteing until the onions are delicate, around 8-10 minutes.

2. Add the bean stew en adobo, the cumin, the stew powder, and the smoked paprika. Warmth until the flavours are incredibly fragrant. Include the tomatoes, dark beans, and vegetable soup.

3. When a stock is foaming, diminish to a stew and cook for roughly 25-30 minutes, or until the sweet potatoes are delicate.

4. Add more stock as required, and season to taste with salt. Serve.

1) Remaining bean stew can be solidified and will keep for as long as five days.

CAULIFLOWER RICE WITH LEMON, MINT, AND PISTACHIOS

Serves 2

Fixings

5 cups crude cauliflower florets

1 oz pistachios

1/4 cup every basil and mint

2 tsp lemon pizzazz

1/2 tbsp lemon juice

1 tbsp olive oil

1/4 cup dried currants

Ocean salt and dark pepper to taste

Technique

1. Port 3 cups of the cauliflower to a nourishment processor. Procedure until the cauliflower is separated into pieces that are about the size of rice. Move to an enormous blending bowl.

2. Transfer staying 2 cups of cauliflower to the nourishment processor. Include the pistachios. The procedure, by and by until cauliflower is separated into rice estimated pieces. Heartbeat in the basil and mint till herbs are finely hacked.

3. Add the extra cleaved cauliflower, pistachios, and herbs to the blending bowl with the central cluster of cauliflower. Include the lemon juice, oil, and flows — season to taste with salt and pepper serve.

DARK COLOURED RICE AND LENTIL SALAD

Serves 4

Fixings

Two tablespoons olive oil

One tablespoon apple juice vinegar

One tablespoon lemon juice

1 tablespoon dijon mustard

1/2 tsp smoked paprika

Ocean salt and dark pepper to taste

2 cups cooked dark coloured rice

1 15-oz can natural, no sodium included lentils, flushed, or 1/cups cooked lentils

One carrot, diced or ground

4 tbsp cleaved crisp parsley

Technique

1. Whisk oil, vinegar, mustard, paprika, lemon juice salt and pepper together in an enormous bowl.

2. Add the rice, lentils, carrot and parsley. Blend well and serve

Crude "Shelled nut" NOODLES

Serves 2

Fixings

For the dressing:

One tablespoon ground ginger

1/2 cup olive oil

2 tsp sesame oil (toasted)

2 tbsp smooth white miso

Three dates, set, or ¼ cup maple syrup

1 tbsp Nama shoyu

1/4 cup water

For the noodles:

2 zucchinis

1 red ringer pepper, cut into matchsticks

1 carrot, ground

1 little cucumber, stripped into flimsy strips

1 cup meagerly cut, steamed snow peas

1/4 cup slashed scallions or green onion

Technique

1. Blend dressing fixings in a fast blender until all fixings are velvety and smooth.

2. Cut the zucchini into long, flimsy "noodles." Combine the carrot with the pepper, zucchini, cucumber, and scallions.

3. Dress the noodles with enough dressing to cover them well. Serve.

SIMPLE FRIED RICE AND VEGETABLES

Serves 2

Fixings

2 tsp toasted sesame oil

1 tbsp ground ginger

1/2 cups cooked darker rice

2-3 cups solidified or crisp vegetables of decision

1 tbsp low sodium tamari

1 tbsp rice vinegar

Vegetable juices as required

Technique

1. Heat the sesame oil in an enormous wok. Include the ground ginger and warmth it for a moment or two.

2. Add the dark coloured rice and vegetables. Saute till the vegetables are delicate.

3. Add the tamari, rice vinegar, and a sprinkle of vegetable stock if the blend is dry. Serve.

ARUGULA SALAD WITH GOJI BERRIES, ROASTED BUTTERNUT SQUASH, AND CAULIFLOWER

Serves 2

Fixings

For the plate of mixed greens:

Four stacking cups arugula (or other green)

1 lb butternut squash, stripped and cleaved

1 little head cauliflower, washed and cleaved into little florets

2 tbsp coconut or olive oil

Ocean salt and pepper to taste

1/4 cup crude pumpkin seeds

1/4 cup goji berries

For the dressing:

3 tbsp olive oil

2 tbsp squeezed orange

1 tbsp lemon juice

1/2 tsp turmeric

1/4 tsp ground ginger

1 tbsp agave or maple syrup

Ocean salt to taste.

Strategy

1. Hurl the cauliflower in the other tablespoon and season with salt and pepper. Broil the two veggies at 375 degrees for 20-

Thirty minutes (the cauliflower will cook quicker), till brilliant darker and fragrant. Expel from the stove and let it cool.

2. Place the goji berries, arugula, and pumpkin seeds in an enormous bowl. Include boiled vegetables. Mix the olive oil, lemon juice, turmeric, maple syrup or agave, ginger together, and ocean salt, and dress every one of the veggies.

3. Divide serving of mixed greens onto two plates, and serve.

COOKED VEGETABLE PESTO PASTA SALAD

Note: Instead of utilizing dark coloured rice or quinoa pasta in this dish, you can likewise blend the cooked vegetables and pesto into an entire grain, similar to darker rice or millet or quinoa, for a progressively healthy variety.

Serves 4

Fixings

3 cups zucchini, cleaved into 3/4" pieces

3 cups eggplant, cleaved into 3/4" pieces

1 enormous Jersey or treasure tomato, cleaved

2 tbsp olive oil or liquefied coconut oil

Ocean salt and dark pepper to taste

8 oz dark coloured rice or quinoa pasta (penne and fusilli function admirably)

1/2 - 2/3 cup pecan pesto (see: dressings)

Technique

1. Preheat your broiler to 400F.

2. Lay the zucchini, eggplant and tomato out on two material or foil fixed heating sheets and shower with the olive or coconut oil. Coat the vegetables with the oil and meal vegetables for thirty minutes, or until delicate and searing.

3. While vegetable cook, carry a pot of salted water to bubble. Include the pasta and cook till still somewhat firm (as per bundle guidelines). Channel pasta and put aside in a considerable blending bowl.

1. Add the cooked vegetables and to the pasta. Blend in the pesto, season to taste, and serve without a moment's delay.

PORTOBELLO "STEAK" AND CAULIFLOWER "Pureed potatoes."

Serves 4

Fixings

For the mushrooms:

1/4 cup olive oil

2 tbsp balsamic vinegar

2 tbsp low sodium tamari or nama shoyu

4 tbsp maple syrup

Sprinkle pepper

4 portobello mushroom tops, cleaned

Submerge 4 Portobello tops in the marinade. 1 hour will be sufficient for them to be prepared, yet medium-term in the refrigerator is stunningly better.

For the Cauliflower Mashed Potatoes:

1 cups cashews, crude

4 cups cauliflower, hacked into little florets and pieces

2 tbsp smooth white miso

3 tbsp healthful yeast

2 tbsp lemon juice

Ocean salt and dark pepper to taste

1/3 cup (or less) water

Technique

1. Place cashews into the bowl of your nourishment processor, and procedure into a fine powder.

2. Add the miso, lemon juice, dietary yeast, pepper, and cauliflower. Heartbeat to join. With the engine of the machine running, include water in a meagre stream, until the blend starts to take on a smooth, whipped surface. You may need to stop much of the time to clean the sides of the bowl and help it along.

3. When the blend takes after pureed potatoes, stop, scoop, and serve close by a Portobello top.

QUINOA ENCHILADAS

Adjusted from a formula in Food52

Serves 6

Fixings

1 tbsp coconut oil

Two cloves garlic, minced

1 little yellow onion, cleaved

3/4 pounds child Bella mushrooms, hacked

1/2 cup diced green bean stews

1/2 teaspoon ground cumin

1/4 teaspoon ocean salt (or to taste)

One can make natural, low sodium dark beans or 1/2 cup cooked dark beans.

1/2 cup cooked quinoa

10 6-inch corn tortillas

1/4 cup natural, low sodium tomato or enchilada sauce

Strategy

1. Preheat stove to 350 degrees.

2. In a hot big pot, warm coconut oil. (around 5-8 min). Include mushrooms and cook until the fluid has been discharged and vanished (another 5 min).

3. Add the bean stews to the pot and give them a mix for 2 minutes. Include the cumin, ocean salt, dark beans, and quinoa, and keep warming the blend until it's hot.

4. Spread a skinny layer (1/2 cup) of marinara or enchilada sauce in the base of a meal dish. Spot 33% of a cup of quinoa blend in the focal point of a corn tortilla and move it up. Spot the tortilla, crease down, in the goulash dish. Rehash with every single residual tortilla and after that spread them with 3/4 cup of extra sauce. Prepare for 25 minutes and serve.

4. SNACK AND DESSERTS RECIPES

SNACKS

HEMP HUMMUS

Serves 4

Fixings

1/4 cup shelled hemp seeds

1 can chickpeas, depleted, or 2 cups newly cooked chickpeas 1/2 tsp salt (to taste)

2-3 tbsp newly pressed lemon juice (to taste)

1 little clove garlic, minced

1 tbsp tahini (discretionary)

1/2 tsp cumin

Water as required

Technique

1. Put the hemp seeds inside the bowl of a nourishment processor and granulate till fine.

2. Add the chickpeas, the salt, the lemon, the garlic, tahini, and cumin, and start to process. Include water in a slight stream (halting to scratch the bowl a couple of times) until the blend is thoroughly smooth and velvety.

3. Garnish with additional hemp seeds and serve. Hummus will keep in the refrigerator for as long as four days

PEANUT BUTTER AND JELLY SNACK BALLS

Makes 20 Balls

Fixings

1/2 cups natural broiled, unsalted peanuts

1/2 cups dull raisins

2 tablespoons nutty spread

Squeeze ocean salt

Strategy

1. Add all fixings to a nourishment processor and procedure till the peanuts are separated and the blend is beginning to remain together. It might discharge a little oil. However, that is OK.

2. Roll blend into 1 inch balls. Store in the ice chest for in any event thirty minutes before serving.

SWEET POTATO HUMMUS

Serves 6

Fixings

2 cups sweet potato, steamed or heated and cut into 3D shapes

1 can natural, low sodium chickpeas, depleted (or 1/2 cups cooked chickpeas)

1/2 tsp sesame oil

1/4 cup tahini

1 tablespoon lemon juice

1/2 tsp smoked paprika

1/2 tsp salt

Dark pepper to taste

1/2 cup water + more as required

Technique

1. Place the sweet potato, the chickpeas, the sesame oil, the tahini, lemon, salt and pepper into a nourishment processor. Heartbeat to join.

2. Turn on the engine and sprinkle in 1/2 water. Procedure blend, halting a couple of times to scratch down the bowl. Include more water as required until you have a velvety, smooth finished hummus. Serve.
DRESSINGS

TURMERIC TAHINI DRESSING

Makes 1/2 Cups

Fixings

1/2 cup tahini

2 tablespoons apple juice vinegar

2 tablespoons coconut aminos or tamari

1/2 teaspoonful of ginger (or 1 teaspoon crisp, ground ginger)

2 teaspoons turmeric

1 teaspoon maple syrup

2/3 - 3/4 cup water

Technique

Mix all fixings in a blender or nourishment processor till smooth. Start with 2/3 cup water and include more as required (dressing will thicken in the ice chest).

Pecan PESTO

Makes 1 liberal cup

Fixings

1 cup coarsely slashed pecans

2 1/2 cups pressed new basil leaves, washed and dried

1 enormous garlic clove

1 tbsp lemon pizzazz

Juice of 1 lemon

1/4 cup wholesome yeast

1/2 cup high additional virgin olive oil

Salt and pepper to taste

Strategy

1. Grind pecans in a nourishment processor till finely ground. Include basil and heartbeat till it frames a coarse blend.

2. Add the garlic, lemon pizzazz and juice, and dietary yeast, and heartbeat a couple of more occasions. Turn the engine on and keep running as you include olive oil in a thin stream. I like my pesto exceptionally thick, however, include more oil on the off chance that you want a more slender blend. Add salt and pepper to taste. Use, or stop as required.

BALSAMIC TAHINI DRESSING

Makes 1/4 cups

Fixings

1/2 cup tahini

1/4 cup balsamic vinegar

1/2 cup water

1/4 teaspoon of garlic powder, or 1/2 clove finely minced garlic 1 tbsp tamari or nama shoyu

Strategy

Mix all fixings in a blender or nourishment processor. Include more water as required.

CRUDE RANCH DRESSING

Makes 1 ½ cups

Fixings

¾ cup cashews, doused for in any event two hours and depleted ½ cup water

2 tbsp lemon juice

¼ cup apple juice vinegar ¼-½ teaspoon salt.

½ tsp dried thyme ½ tsp dried oregano 1 clove garlic

3 tbsp new dill

3 tbsp new parsley

3 tbsp olive oil

Strategy

Mix all fixings in a rapid blender and serve.

Smooth APRICOT GINGER DRESSING

Makes about 2 cups (formula can be divided)

INGREDIENTS

1/2 cup dried apricots, stuffed

3/4 inch long handle crude ginger (or 1/2 tsp ginger powder)

1/2 cup squeezed orange

1/2 cup water

2 tbsp apple juice vinegar

1 tbsp tamari or nama shoyu

2 tbsp olive oil

Strategy

Mix all dressing fixings in a rapid blender and serve.

Fig and White Balsamic Vinaigrette

Makes 1/4 cups

Fixings

6 exceptionally huge dried figs (if yours are little, include a couple of increasingly), drenched for around 8 hours and depleted

1/3 white balsamic vinegar (subordinary if need be)

1/4 cup olive oil

1/4 water

1 little clove garlic

1 tbsp dijon mustard

Salt and dark pepper to taste

Technique

Mix all fixings in an electric blender till absolutely smooth and creamy. Include more water if it's excessively thick.

DESSERTS

BANANA SOFT SERVE

Makes 2 servings

Fixings

2 huge bananas, stripped and hacked into pieces, at that point solidified 1/2 teaspoon vanilla

Strategy

Spot bananas in a nourishment processor and turn the engine on. Give the processor a chance to keep running until the bananas have gotten progressively light, soft, and smooth. They'll take after a creamy bowl of delicate serve frozen yoghurt!

You may need to stop a couple of times to scratch the bowl down. Be patient and let the processor carry out its responsibility — from the start it'll appear as if the delicate serve isn't meeting up. However, it will. Present with any fixings you like: cacao nibs, dim chocolate, nutty spread, cleaved nuts or seeds

CRUDE VEGAN BROWNIE BITES

Makes 24-30 balls

Fixings

2 cups pecans

2/3 cup cacao nibs

Liberal squeeze ocean salt (to taste)

1/4 cup crude cacao (or ordinary cocoa) powder

1/2 cups set dates

Strategy

1. Place the pecans, cacao nibs, ocean salt, and cacao powder in a nourishment processor and procedure for some times, or till everything is truly very much crushed up.

2. Add the dates and procedure for an additional twenty seconds or somewhere in the vicinity. The blend ought to stay together. If it's not, continue handling until it stays together effectively when you press a little in your grasp. If you have to, including a couple of more dates will help tie it together.

3. Shape the "mixture" into balls that are around 3/4 - 1 inch thick by moving it in your palms. Store in the refrigerator for 30 minutes, and after that, they'll be prepared to serve.

1. Balls will keep, put away in the cooler, for about fourteen days.

CRUDE, VEGAN VANILLA MACAROONS

Makes 15 macaroons

Fixings

1/2 cup crude almonds

One piling cup unsweetened destroyed coconut

1/4 cup coconut oil (will be most straightforward to move up the macaroons if the oil is healthy when you placed it in the processor)

Three tablespoons maple syrup

1 teaspoon vanilla concentrate

Squeeze ocean salt

Strategy

1. Add almonds to the nourishment processor and procedure till they're finely ground.

2. Add the rest of the fixings and procedure once more, till everything is very much consolidated.

3. Working rapidly (or else the coconut oil will soften) fold the coconut blend into little (3/4" - 1") balls — spot on a material lined platter or heating sheet.

4. Transfer platter to the ice chest, and refrigerate for a couple of hours, till the macaroons are strong. Serve.

Macaroons will keep in the refrigerator for as long as about fourteen days.

CHOCOMOLE

Serves 2

Fixings

1 huge, ready Haas avocado, set

½ tsp vanilla

4 piling tablespoons crude cacao powder

3 tbsp maple syrup or agave

1/4 cup water (more as required)

Strategy

Spot all fixings in a nourishment processor or Vitamix and mix till smooth. Serve.

BLUEBERRY GINGER ICE CREAM

Serves 2

Fixings

2 solidified bananas

1 piling cup solidified blueberries

1/2 inch new ginger (or 1/2 tsp ginger powder in case you're utilizing a nourishment processor)

1/4 cup cashews

2 tsp lemon juice

2-4 tbsp almond or hemp milk

Strategy

Mix all fixings in a rapid blender. Begin with 3 tbsp of almond milk and utilize the pack to attempt to get the blend moving without including an excessive amount of fluid: you need a frozen yoghurt, not a smoothie! If you need the additional two tablespoons, use them, yet be patient and continue mixing with the pack till a thick consistency is accomplished.

#PLANT BASED DIET FOR SUCCESS

CUSTOM MADE HEMP SEED MILK

INSTRUCTION MAKE HEMP MILK

A fast and simple 2-fixing, brief approach to make natively constructed hemp milk! Normally velvety and sweet, and ideal for smoothies, granola, and the sky is the limit from there!

PREP TIME5 minutes

Complete TIME5 minutes

Servings: (1/2-cup servings)

Class: Beverage

Cooking: Gluten-Free, Vegan

Cooler Friendly multi month

Does it keep? 5 Days

Fixings

- 1/2 cup hemp seeds

- 3-4 cups water (utilize less water for thicker, creamier milk!)

- 1 squeeze ocean salt

- 1 entire date, set (discretionary/for sweetness/or 1 Tbsp (15 ml) maple syrup)

- 1/2 tsp vanilla concentrate (discretionary)

- 2 tablespoon ocoa or cacao powder for "chocolate milk" (discretionary)

- 1/4 cup 1/4 cup new berries for "berry milk" (discretionary)

Directions

1.   Add hemp seeds, water, salt, and any extra include ins (discretionary) to a rapid blender. Top with top and spread with a towel to guarantee it doesn't sprinkle. Mix for around 1 moment or until the blend appears to be very much joined.

2.   Scoop out a little example with a spoon to test flavor/sweetness. Include more dates, salt, or vanilla as required.

3.   Pour the blend legitimately into a serving compartment. You can strain it. However, it needn't bother with it, I would say. If stressing, pour over an enormous blending bowl or pitcher secured with a nut milk sack, slender towel, or a perfect T-shirt.

4.   Transfer to a fixed compartment and refrigerate. Protect it in the freezer for as long as 5 days (in some cases more). Appreciate cold (and shake well) for the best outcomes. It's delightful directly from the container, in smoothies, with granola, or in heated products.

FLUID NUTRITION SMOOTHIE
Prep time: 4 min • Yield: 3 servings

2 cups rice milk, 2 almond milk, 2 to 4 tablespoons plant-based protein powder, (for example, Sunwarrior or Vega) ½ cup blueberries or blended berries, new or solidified 1 banana ½ cup slashed mango, peach, or pear, crisp or solidified ½ cup ice 1 teaspoon coconut nectar or crude

nectar ½ to 1 cup pressed new spinach leaves 1 Blend every one of the fixings in a blender until the blend is smooth and no protuberances remain. 2 Pour into two glasses and appreciate it.

Fixings Directions

Per serving: Calories 186 (From Fat 27); Fat 4g (Saturated 0g); Cholesterol 0mg; Sodium 284mg; Carbohydrate 31g (Dietary Fiber 4g); Protein 11g. Note: The smoothie will keep for eight hours in the icebox. Change It! Take a stab at including a tbspn of any of these superfoods: goji berries, cacao nibs, coconut oil, flax oil, chia seeds, hempseeds, carob powder, maca, matcha green-tea powder, almond margarine, or acai-berry powder.

Tip: This smoothie will be creamier if your fruit is solidified, so choose solidified fruit at whatever point conceivable (or include more ice).

BLUEBERRY BUCKWHEAT PANCAKES
Prep time: 10 min •

Cook time: 25 min

• Yield: 4–6 servings

1 In a little bowl, join the buckwheat flour, heating powder, salt, preparing pop, and precious maple stones. Put in a safe spot.

2 In an enormous bowl, join the apple-juice vinegar and rice milk. Let's sit for 5 to 15 minutes, at that point, include the pounded banana.

3 Add the dry fixings to the wet fixings. Beat distinctly until mixed.

4 Add the blueberries. 5 Heat the coconut oil on an iron. Utilizing a 1-ounce spoon, pour the player onto the lubed iron. Cook the flapjacks until the air pockets in the hitter break superficially; flip and cook until carmelized. Rehash until you're out of the player.

6 Serve on plate and top it with the maple syrup, cinnamon, crisp fruit, coconut yogurt, or cashew cream.

Fixings Directions

Per serving: Calories 349 (From Fat 63); Fat 7g (Saturated 3g); Cholesterol 0mg; Sodium 701mg; Carbohydrate 65g (Dietary Fiber 10g); Protein 12g. Change It! Attempt these flapjacks with various fruits, for example, cranberries or strawberries, or make them significantly progressively wanton by including some non-dairy chocolate chips. You can likewise substitute another without gluten or entire grain flour, for example, dark colored rice or oat flour for the buckwheat flour.

APPLE CINNAMON MINI-MUFFINS
Preparation time: 30 min

• Cook time: 15 min

• Yield: 12–20 small scale biscuits

1 cup spelt flour, kamut flour, or oat flour ½ cup moved oats 1 teaspoon heating powder ½ teaspoon preparing soft drink ¼ teaspoon cinnamon ¼ teaspoon ocean salt ¼ cup coconut oil or grapeseed oil ¼ cup maple syrup 1/3 cup fruit purée ½ cup rice milk 1 apple, seeded and cut into little blocks ½ cup raisins 1 Preheat the stove to 350 degrees. 2 Combine the dry fixings in an enormous bowl. Put in a safe spot. 3 Combine the wet fixings and apples in a medium bowl. 4 Pour the wet fixings into the dry fixings and blend well, ensuring there are no bumps. Mix in the raisins. 5 Distribute the blend equitably in a 24-cup smaller than normal biscuit dish. You can utilize coconut oil or grapeseed oil to oil the tin, or use paper liner cups. 6 Bake for 12 minutes. 7 Remove the skillet from the stove and let it sit for a few moments; at that point, expel the biscuits and cool them on a cooling rack or plate.

Fixings Directions

Per serving: Calories 140 (From Fat 45); Fat 5g (Saturated 4g); Cholesterol 0mg; Sodium 115mg; Carb 23g (Dietary Fiber 2g); Protein 2g. Note: Be certain to utilize unbleached material paper cups. These are dark colored, not white. You don't need any buildup draining into your delectable biscuits! Differ It! Utilize this recipe to make 8 to 12 full-sized biscuits —make certain to stretch out the heating time to 20 minutes. You can likewise swap in a sans gluten flour, for example, dark colored rice flour. Tip: If you have void biscuit cups after filling the cups with the player, add water to the vacant cups to avoid consuming.

MORNING MILLET GRANOLA
Prep time: 8 min • Cook time: 25 min • Yield: Approx 6 cups

¾ cup unadulterated natural maple syrup 1 tablespoon rice milk ¼ cup coconut oil 4 cups moved oats 1½ cups puffed millet oat or millet drops ¾ cup sesame seeds ½ cup sunflower seeds ½ cup pumpkin seeds 1 cup unsweetened coconut chips ¼ cup flaxseeds 1 cup cleaved almonds 1 teaspoon ocean salt 1½ cups raisins, apricots, or cranberries (unsulphured) 1 Preheat the broiler to 300 degrees. 2 Combine the 2 maple syrup, rice milk and coconut oil in an enormous pot and put in a safe spot. 3 Mix the rest of the fixings, except the raisins, in an enormous bowl. Hurl well. 4 Add the syrup blend and mix well. 5 Pour the blend into two shallow skillet or preparing sheets fixed with material paper and heat for 15 minutes. Mix, at that point, heat for an extra 10 minutes. 6 Take the granola out of the broiler and include the raisins. 7 Cool and store in a hermetically sealed compartment.

Fixings

Per serving: Calories 282 (From Fat 117); Fat 14g (Cholesterol 0mg; Sodium 73mg; Carbohydrate 42g (Dietary Fiber 5g); Protein 5g. Note: Don't include the raisins or other dried fruits too soon — they get exceptionally hard whenever heated in the stove. Differ It! Rather than millet, you can utilize oat grain, quinoa, or amaranth chips. Tip: Serve this granola with coconut yogurt and top it with new berries for a generous breakfast enchant. Note: Be certain that the dried fruit you purchase is sulphite free. Suphates are additives that keep fruit "new" long after it has been collected. Continuously check to ensure the dried fruit you purchase is free of this added substance.

Drenched Oats with Goji Berries

Prep time: 10 min in addition to drenching time • Cook time: 2–10 min • Yield: 1–2 servings

Fixings

Entire moved oats ½ cup water 1 tablespoon new pressed lemon juice ½ cup rice milk or almond milk 1 tablespoon almond margarine 1 banana, cut 2 tablespoons goji berries 1 teaspoon cinnamon ¼ cup pumpkin seeds 1 tablespoon maple syrup 1 Combine the oats, water, and lemon squeeze in a bowl. Spread with a plate and drench medium-term at room temperature. 2 For cold oats, add the rest of the fixings to the bowl and appreciate. 3 For warm oats, add every one of the fixings to a pot with an extra sprinkle of rice milk. Warm for 5 minutes and serve.

OTHER PLANT BASED RECIPES

Vegan Mushroom Tetrazzini
Another go-to family dinner including your favored things: Hungarian Mushroom Soup, and Mama's Mac Sauce. This smooth, flavorful extraordinary will make you dismiss consistently using

cheddar in a goulash again. It's stacked with protein, potassium, and safety boosting micronutrients!

Prep time: 15 minutes

Warmth time: 45 minutes

Servings: 8

Fixings:

1 pack of Hungarian Mushroom Soup

1 pack of Mama's Mac Sauce

Dull hued rice lasagna noodles or no-prepare sans gluten noodles

8oz of mushrooms1 clove of garlic

1 Tablespoon of parsley

Squashed dull pepper

4 cups of separated spinach

Cooking Instructions:

Saute... Mushrooms in a little water until fragile. By then, incorporate garlic and parsley and cook for an extra 3 minutes.

Layer in a grill safe meal dish...

Layer 1: 1/4 a pack of MamaSezz Hungarian Mushroom Soup

Layer 2: Noodles

Layer 3: 1/4 a pack of MamaSezz Hungarian Mushroom Soup

Layer 4: Your cooked mushrooms

Layer 5: 1/3 a pack of Mama's Mac Sauce

Layer 6: Noodles

Layer 7: 1/4 a pack of Hungarian Mushroom Soup

Layer 8: Spinach

Layer 9: 1/3 a pack of Mama's Mac Sauce

Layer 10: Noodles

Layer 11: 1/4 a pack of Hungarian Mushroom Soup

Layer 12: 1/3 a pack of plant diet Mama's Mac Sauce

Dairy Free Pumpkin Spiced Latte
Time to take out your woolen garments and agreeable socks since it's pumpkin flavor season! It's definitely not hard to disdain on, look into amusingly, and a while later end up venerating. Here is a plant-based pumpkin get-up-and-go latte recipe that is creamier than the real thing! No keeping things under control in line for a Starbucks pumpkin spiced latte either. This structure is stacked with protein, fiber, and potassium. It's unprecedented for your skin, and far superior for your gut prosperity. An over the top measure of pumpkin pizzazz never hurt anyone...

Prep Time: 5 minutes (notwithstanding drenching medium-term)

Servings: 1

Fixings:

¼ a cup of cashews

4 dates

½ teaspoons vanilla concentrate

2 Tablespoons pumpkin

2 teaspoons pumpkin get-up-and-go mix

Run of sea salt

1 cup of non-dairy milk

A sprinkle of cinnamon

Cooking Instructions:

Medium-term... Soak your cashews and set dates. Didn't prepare? Ingest them high temp water for at any rate 15 minutes.

Combine... the rest of the fixings beside the cinnamon, until smooth.

Finish with... A sprinkle of cinnamon or a cinnamon stick if you're feeling bubbly.

Optional: incorporate a sprinkle of coffee for morning support.

Chewy Oatmeal Banana Pancakes: Vegan and Gluten Free

These without gluten, vegan banana hotcakes will overpower you. Time to bring back Sunday early lunch the right way! They're not hard to prepare, squeezed with potassium, calcium, fiber, and plant protein. Strong, clear, and great for the whole family-It's that easy to eat right.

Cook time: 10 minutes for each cake

Prep time: 10 minutes

Servings: 8 hotcakes

Fixings:

1 ½ cups of without gluten oats

1 cup of unsweetened non-dairy milk

3 Tablespoons of chia seeds

6 dates

3 prepared bananas (the riper, the better!)

1 teaspoon of cinnamon

A run of sea salt

Cooking Instructions:

Combine in a sustenance processor… 1 cup of oats, plant based milk, chia seeds, dates, 2 bananas, cinnamon and sea salt. Blend until smooth.

Vegan Dessert Sauce: Chocolate and Vanilla

Despite whether you eat refined sugars or not this plant-based recipe will make sure to change your dessert game forever.

Use it as a cake coat, hotcake syrup, oatmeal besting, a cupcake icing, even as a pudding. Dunk strawberries in it on your recognition… or a treat-yo-self Tuesday night! This sound embellishment is loaded down with nutrients, so why limit yourself to just one gathering?

Prep time: 5 Minutes (notwithstanding medium-term splashing)

Servings: 4 servings

Fixings

1/2 cup of rough cashews, splashed

8 dates, drenched

1/8 tsp of sea salt

1 Tablespoons of cacao

Rules

The earlier night... Absorb cashews and dates water

(Didn't prepare? Me either. Retain cashews and dates high temp water for around 15 minutes until fragile)

At the point when doused, combine... Cashews, dates, and sea salt

Mix into half (optional)... **Cacao Powder**

Strong Spicy Watermelon Summer Salad Recipe
Summer is here, and child did it please strong. For sure, even New Englanders are breaking out the cooling. The best way to deal with beat the glow? This fiery watermelon summer is serving of blended greens recipe. It's restoring, excellent, and perfect for drawing in - notwithstanding the way that it is brilliant.

Cook time: 0 minutes

Prep time: 5 minutes

Fixings

Watermelon

Lime Juice

Sea Salt

Fresh mint

Peanuts

Cayenne Pepper

Rules

First... Cut watermelon into bumps (be careful!)

By then, incorporate... Only a little press of sea salt (or skirt the salt!)

Spritz with... Some fresh lime juice

Sprinkle with... Vegan Sour Cream

Sprinkle with...Peanuts (rough or stewed)

Buildup with... Just a spot of cayenne pepper

In conclusion, top with... New mint

Plant-Based Side Dish: Garlic Ginger Broccoli

There's clarification watchman control their adolescents to eat broccoli... it has astonishing medicinal points of interest! In any case, this plant-based side dish isn't your mother's steamed broccoli recipe, and trust me, and you won't have to drive anyone to eat it. The puzzle? The garlic ginger sauce. Sweet, salty and red hot - extraordinary to indisputably the last eat. Prepare a meal out of it by eating it over darker rice with a side serving of blended greens or near to your favored vegan smoothie.

Prep Time: 5 minutes

Prep Time: 15 minutes

Servings: 2-4

Fixings:

1 head of broccoli, chop into diminished down pieces

2 cloves of garlic, minced

1 TBSP of ginger, minced

2 TBSP of low sodium Tamari

2 TBSP of nectar or agave

1 (+) TBSP of bean stew stick (incorporate more for heat)

1 TBSP of sesame seeds

Headings:

1.   Sauté broccoli in several TBS of water, until broccoli begins to turn splendid green, around 5-8 minutes. Incorporate more water when required.

2.   Put the broccoli to the sides of the dish, and in the inside sauté the garlic and ginger until it gets fragrant around 2-5 minutes.

3.   Once ginger and garlic are cooked, incorporate the rest of the fixings to the point of convergence of the dish and join. At the point when joined, mix into broccoli.

4.   Cook and reduce it, until broccoli is at a perfect delicacy, and the sauce has gotten thick and tenacious.

5.   Enjoy hot

Youngster Friendly Plant-Based Breakfast Panini Recipe

Who says sandwiches must be a choice meal? This chocolate, cinnamon, nutty spread panini will cause them to eat outside of the case. Likewise, it a fantastic youngster genial plant-based breakfast. With unquestionably no refined sugar or included sugar, this vegan meal is squeezed with fiber, protein, potassium, and malignant growth anticipation operators.

Prep Time: 5 minutes

Yield: 1

Fixings:

¼ cup of raisins

¼ cup of warmed water

1 TBSP cinnamon

2 tsp cacao powder

¼ cup of trademark nutty spread

1 prepared banana

2 cuts of whole grain bread

Headings:

1. Mix raisins, warmed water, cinnamon, and cacao powder

2. Spread nutty spread on whole grain bread

3. Slice banana and store onto nutty spread toast

4. Blend raisin mix, and spread into a sandwich

No-Cook Vegan Lemon Cheesecake

A whole sustenance plant-based lifestyle doesn't mean saying goodbye to your favored sustenance, like dessert. This sound turn on vegan lemon cheesecake is totally licked the fork, lick the plate, return for a seriously long time and do it again, gooood. It's a no-cook recipe (perfect for warm atmosphere) and 100% refined sugar free!

Prep Time: 20 minutes + medium-term cooling and drenching

Cook Time: 0 minutes

Yield: 10 cuts

Fixings

2 cups of cashews (drench medium-term)

20 Medjool dates (drench 10 medium-term)

1 cup almond meal

½ cup pecans

1 ½ lemons, notwithstanding style

1 Tablespoon flaxseed

2 Tablespoons ground chia seed

1 teaspoon customary vanilla remove

1 Tablespoon stimulating yeast

¼ teaspoon of turmeric

Sea salt to taste

Headings

1. Heartbeat 10 dates (not sprinkled), almond meal, pecans and a run of sea salt in the sustenance processor until split up

2. Press nut and date mix into the base of a pie dish until if structures a firm covering.

3. Blend the rest of the fixings in a blender until smooth

4. Use a spatula to spread it into the most noteworthy purpose of the pie dish

5. Chill medium-term and appreciate

Dairy-Free Potato Leek Soup Recipe

This sans dairy potato leek soup is the perfect lovely answer for your comfort sustenance longings. Besides, with only 8 fixings and concise cook time, you can benefit as much as possible from your solid vegan comfort sustenance sooner rather than later...preferably with a conventional book and your favored hurl spread.

Prep Time: 5-10 minutes

Cook Time: 25 minutes

Yield: 4-5 servings

Fixings

2 clove garlic, diced

Two leeks, diced

4 Yukon Gold potatoes, hacked

2 ribs celery, hacked

4 cups veggie soup

2 cups of water

1/2 cup energizing yeast

4 cups of kale or spinach pepper to taste

Cooking Instructions

Saute for 3 minutes in a soup pot over medium heat...

Leeks, celery, and garlic notwithstanding a little water

Add by then bring to a boil...Potatoes, veggie stock, and water.

Decrease to stew and cover for 20 minutes then...Check to check whether potatoes are sensitive.

In case they are, blend...

A huge portion of the soup until smooth. You can use a dousing blender OR spoon a huge portion of the soup into your blender by then add back to the pot when rich.

Blend in until wilted...Spinach and also kale and blend until shriveled.

Finally...Add healthy yeast and serve.

Whole Food Plant Based Cookout Recipe: Mediterranean Potato Salad
Are you Looking for a whole sustenance plant-based excursion recipe? This sans oil potato serving of blended greens will fulfill everyone at the BBQ. Reward: The without dairy mayo recipe can in like manner be used on sandwiches, in dives, and when else you need a mayo replacer.

Remember: You never need to give up your old top decisions when you transition to a plant-based eating routine… essentially modify them :)

Cook Time: 6 minutes

Prep Time: 15 minutes

Servings: 8 servings

Recipe Category: side dish

Fixings

Potato Salad

4 cups of newborn child potatoes (of any arrangement), diced into gigantic pieces

1 cup of dull olives (canned, set)

1 cup of green olives (canned, set)

¼ cup of stunts

1 compartment of artichoke hearts, washed and diced

½ teaspoon of oregano

3 Tablespoons of balsamic vinegar

Whole Food Plant-Based Mayo

1 prepared avocado

½ teaspoon of sea salt

½ teaspoon of garlic powder

1 Tablespoon lemon juice

1 Tablespoon Dijon

a run of dim pepper

several Tablespoons of water

Cooking Instructions

Air pocket until sensitive… Potatoes with essentially enough water to cover (4-6 minutes)

Meanwhile, combine… All the sans dairy mayo fixings

Chop into diminished down pieces… .Artichoke hearts

Join in a significant bowl… .Hot cooked potatoes, sans dairy mayo, vinegar, and oregano

Finally, add…Olives, capers, and artichokes until all mixed in

Vegan Quinoa Lunch Bowl with Broccoli and Mushrooms
A strong vegan lunch bowl that will truly finish you off? You betcha. This Vegan Quinoa Lunch Bowl recipe has a ton of plant-based protein and fiber to keep you full and perky for the duration of the afternoon. Expert tip: bundle cooks this quinoa lunch bowl and store in the fridge for moment meals reliably.

Prep Time: 10 minutes

Cook Time: 30 minutes

Servings: 2

Class: Lunch

Fixings

2 cups of mushrooms, cut

1 head of broccoli, cut

2 immense lots of spinach

1 cup of quinoa, cooked

⅓ teaspoon of garlic powder

½ teaspoon of low sodium tamari

½ teaspoon of lemon juice

1-2 cups of veggie juices

¼ a cup of tahini

Cooking Instructions

In a warmed skillet, saute… Mushrooms and veggie soup until mushrooms are fragile

By then incorporate in…Chopped broccoli and a sprinkle more veggie juices to keep from remaining

At the point when the broccoli's casual, blend in… Cooked quinoa, flavors, Tamari, lemon juice, and spinach.

Right when spinach is wilted… Spoon everything into your favored bowl and shower with tahini

Oil-Free Vegan Fried Rice Recipe

It's the clear things in life…like this magnificent without oil vegan singed rice. Prepared in a brief span, this plant-based dish is a family most cherished hence darn easy to make.

Expert tips

- o   This is a perfect whole sustenance plant-based recipe for group cooking! Make a significant gathering at the start of the week and store in the cooler or the cooler for straightforward sound lunches all through the whole week.

- o   Bulk this vegan scorched rice up with different plant-based protein sources, as prepared tofu, edamame, or chickpeas.

- o Use this recipe as a way to deal with experience the produce in your cooler! You don't have to hold fast to the recipe unequivocally. Any veggies will do. Incorporate broccoli, zucchini, peppers, scallions, pineapple pieces, whatever you have!

Cook Time: 15 minutes

Prep Time: 10 minutes

Servings: 2

Recipe Category: dinner

Fixings

1 onion, diced

Several Tablespoons of veggie stock

2 cloves of garlic, minced

2 cups of hardened peas and carrots

2 cups of cooked dim shaded rice (unmistakably cooked the earlier day)

5 Tablespoons of tamari

Cooking Instructions

Saute over medium heat until sensitive (around 8 minutes)

Diced onion in veggie stock

By then, incorporate… Garlic and blend

Following 1 minute, throw in...

Cooked rice, veggies, and Tamari

Marinara Alla Mama Vegan Pasta Dish

Is your weeknight dinner routine getting stale, or would you say you require a lively (yet unrestrained) vegan pasta dish for a night out on the town? Prepare this debased and straightforward whole sustenance plant-based meal in less than 20 minutes.

Cook Time: 13 minutes

Prep Time: 5 minutes

Servings: 2

Recipe Category: Dinner

Fixings:

2 plant based diet Veggie Sausage patties

1 cup of plant based diet Marinara Sauce

¼ lb of dry whole grain pasta (whole wheat, darker rice, lentil, bean, quinoa)

Cooking Instructions

Add to foaming water

¼ of a pound of dry whole sustenance plant-based pasta of choice and cook until still to some degree firm (check pasta group for express cook times)

While pasta's cooking, heat…

Crumbled pre-cooked Veggie Sausages and mix in with Marinara Sauce

THE USEFULNESS OF PLANT-BASED DIET TO LOSE WEIGHT QUICKLY

Plant-Based Diet is an eating routine considering nourishments gotten from plants, including vegetables, whole grains, vegetables, and characteristic items, in any case, with few or no animal things. The usage of the articulation has changed after some time, and delineations can be found in the articulation "Plant-Based Diet" being used to suggest veggie darling eating regimens, which contain no sustenance from animal sources to vegan eats fewer carbs which consolidate eggs and dairy. Notwithstanding, no meat and to abstains from food with fluctuating number of flying creature based nourishments, for instance, semi-veggie sweetheart weight control plans which contain little proportions of meat.

Numerous people who live on a plant-based diet are thought to remove on money related need.

What Are The Best Sources Of Plant Protein?

Quinoa

Most grains have a little protein, be that as it may, quinoa—actually, a seed—is exceptional it has 8 grams for each glass, including all of the nine essential amino.

Nuts and nut margarine

All nuts contain both strong fats and protein, making them a productive bit of a plant-based diet.

Beans

There are different collections of beans—dull, white, pinto, inheritance, etc. Be that as it may, one thing they all have in like way is their high proportions of protein.

Chickpeas

Generally called garbanzo beans, these vegetables can be prepared into servings of blended greens, fricasseed and salted as a crisp snack, or pureed into a hummus.

Medical advantages of Plant-Based Diet

1.   Lower Blood Pressure

A large number of individuals living a plant-based diet normally have cut down circulatory strain due to a higher affirmation of potassium-rich nourishments.

2.   Lower Cholesterol

Discussing lower cholesterol, it's one of the guideline benefits you'll get from getting a handle on plant-based sustenances. Parcels individuals don't have the foggiest thought regarding that plant contain NO cholesterol.

3.   Better Blood Sugar

The fundamental way to deal with fight high glucose is to eat more fiber. It backs off the absorption of sugars in the dissemination framework, and as needs can help improve how hungry you are for the day.

4.   Lower Rates of Cancer

A low fat, whole sustenances plant-based diet is the primary way to deal with improving your chances of keeping up a vital good way from development risks.

5.   Weight decrease

It is a nourishment high in unrefined; clean whole food sources can improve your odds at getting fit as a fiddle significantly more, in spite of the way that cooked nourishments may help with supplement ingestion.

What Does Plant-Based Diet Mean?

A plant-based diet is an eating regimen from plants, including vegetables, whole grains, vegetables, and common items, anyway with few or no animal things. The usage of the articulation has changed after some time, and outlines can be found in the articulation "plant-based eating schedule" being used to imply veggie darling weight control plans, which contain no nourishment from animal sources to vegan counts calories which fuse eggs and dairy. Be that as it may, no meat, and to abstains from food with contrasting proportions of animal based sustenances, for instance, semi-veggie darling weight control plans which contain little proportions of meat.

25 EXCLUSIVE VEGETARIAN RECIPES IDEAS FOR HEALTHY WEIGHT LOSS

Eating in night time won't make you include weight, regardless, eating bunches of nourishment that causes you to outperform your step by step calorie confirmation will. If you have to drop pounds, endeavor this technique: make vegetarian recipes a piece of lunch and breakfast, and have less during dinner. Eating such a great amount before a light dinner promises you have sufficient opportunity to devour every last one of those calories.

25 Best Vegetarian Recipes Ideas for Weight Loss

Discover the Reasons That Make You Love With Vegetarian Weight Loss Diet! before you uncover the best vegetarian recipes.

Garlic Mushrooms

You can incorporate various herbs as well, for instance, rosemary, oregano or even fairly hacked mint. This vegetarian recipe is low splashed fat, low carb, low sugar, and low sodium.

Cooked Sweet Potato and Black Bean Burrito

Cooked sweet potatoes spinning with sensitive dim beans and corn, succulent red peppers, and heavenly tomatoes enclosed by a warm whole wheat tortilla make this one magnificent and fulfilling feast.

Cauliflower Crust Pizza

Attempt this Cauliflower Crust Pizza. Freshly ground cauliflower fills in as the base for the innovative and heavenly structure that you can cover up just like customary pizza!

Low Fat Cheesy Stuffed Mushrooms

Mushrooms are one of the superfoods in vegetarian recipes. They're low in calories, sugar, and salt, without fat, cholesterol free, and are a basic wellspring of fiber. Mushrooms are similarly one of just a bunch couple of typical wellsprings of nutrient D, which is crucial for strong bones and teeth.

Gluten-Free Cheesy Veggie "Pasta" Bake

If you needn't bother with gluten, you can even now value this gooey pasta dish. It isn't produced using sans gluten pasta! It is a finished result of spaghetti squash and tremendous measures of other awesome veggies.

Potato, Capsicum, Mushroom Frittata

Mushrooms are high in fiber, low in sugars, calories and sodium and are cholesterol and without fat while capsicum, which is stacked with nutrients A, C, and beta carotene, is also typically low in fat, calories, and cholesterol.

Cauliflower "Rice" Stir-Fry

This Cauliflower "Rice" Stir-Fry has zero cholesterol, is low in sodium, and offers your body nutrient An and nutrient C in just a single meal.

Chicken and Mushroom Risotto

Chicken and Mushroom Risotto is an extraordinarily acclaimed vegetarian recipe. It should take around 30 minutes to make and can be warmed in a microwave the next day, just incorporate a little water before microwaving.

Polenta and Beans

This turn on the fundamental burrito is aggregate without gluten. Instead of being enveloped by a flour tortilla, the delectable beans, and a veggie mix is served over sautéed polenta.

Spaghetti in addition to Spinach - White Wine Garlic Sauce

New make, and a fragrant white wine and garlic sauce keep this veggie sweetheart recipe low in calories yet plentiful in flavor and enhancements like nutrients An and C. Best your dish with a couple of cuts of warmed tofu.

Smooth Chicken Pappardelle

Pappardelle pasta is wide strip pasta that holds sauce on its surface incredibly well. In any case be forewarned, a little runs far with this pasta which is very filling. This Vegan recipe has low sugar, low fat, and high protein.

Sweet Potato, Chickpea, and Quinoa Veggie Burger

It is the best among all vegetarian recipes and less requesting to make than you may speculate. This chickpea, quinoa veggie burger is prepared with warmed sweet potato, cumin, and fresh parsley.

Veggie darling Split Pea Plus Sweet Potato Soup

Appreciate this mouth-watering, smooth, and liberal, customary split pea. You can neglect a lot of a stretch dispose of the meat and prepare the soup with sweet potatoes for a delicious vegetarian bend.

Quick Creamy Chicken and Broccoli Bake

This dish has significance and paying little mind to the likelihood that the youths couldn't care less for broccoli, substitute with peas and corn, cauliflower or even zucchini and mushrooms.

Moderate Cooker Beef and Vegetables

It should be nothing unforeseen that this dish tastes so shocking when you look at the fixings summary and see things like garlic, pumpkin, Worcestershire sauce, Balsamic vinegar, capsicum, smoked paprika, and onions.

Low-Calorie Spinach Soup

You will inside and out value this enhancement thick, easy to design spinach soup. Cooking utilizing low-fat channel proffers it an immaculate emerald green shading with the smell of sautéed onions together with garlic, which makes the soup scrumptious!

Low Fat Paneer

Low fat paneer delivered utilizing low-fat channel, and low-fat curds contain more protein and calcium than full fat paneer. This equation yields one proportion of ground, deteriorated or cubed paneer.

Flax Seeds with Curd and Honey

Enormous portions of us think about the therapeutic favorable circumstances of flax seeds, be that as it may, are at a mishap how to consolidate it into our eating schedule. It considers seed is a fortune trove of omega-3 unsaturated fats, which assist offset with excursion cell dividers and reduce exacerbation.

Mixed Sprouts Fruits and Veggie Salad

Be set up for a challenging foundation squeezed into a plate of blended greens bowl! The Mixed Sprouts Fruits and Veggie Salad has a minor piece of everything, giving your feeling of taste a powerful undertaking, with different flavors and surfaces.

Tomato Methi Rice

Blend methi greens with nutrient c rich tomatoes which help in the ingestion of iron. For an additional fiber contact, use the unpolished dull shaded rice.

Green Pea Parathas

Parathas are keeping up and sound nourishment. Blend puréed green peas with whole wheat flour to make this superb paratha blend. Both the whole wheat flour and the green peas are wealthy in fiber, which aides in controlling glucose levels.

Nutty Spread Coconut Balls

In the event that you pass by this yummy baked good without tasting it, at that point there is a significant issue with your sweet tooth! You can make it by nutty spread and coconut with a run of cocoa. Evaporated the coconut to get a flaky surface and overwhelming visual intrigue.

Dull hued Bread

Who can contradict a cut of fresh warm bread dissipated with nectar? Along these lines, with minor fixings, this Brown Bread recipe is a shot way to deal with making choice, low-calorie wheat bread at home.

Energetic Vegetable Broth

Energetic Vegetable Broth gives heaps of vitality and enhancements while in like manner being amazingly alleviating and pleasant, to such a degree, that it sends a warm feeling through you, loosening up your nerves as you take every spoonful.

Solid Sheera

Solid sheera is stacked with supplements. Whole wheat flour and soy are three flours that are protein rich, while almonds and jaggery incorporate press.

Pumpkin Soup

You would never have imagined the probability of preparing such a lavish soup at a low-calorie count. Thickened with a mix of a low-fat channel, this Pumpkin Soup clears out the necessity for cream yet at the same time holds the excellent smoothness.

#A Plant-Based Diet Can Reduce Your Risk for Type 2 Diabetes, If You Do It Correctly

Specialists state not all plant-based eating regimens are the equivalent. They offer explicit exhortation on the best way to benefit from your nourishment plans. Crisp vegetables are a decent decision. Some prepared plant-based nourishments aren't generally the best choice. Getty Images. Type 2 diabetes is definitely more entangled than basically having eaten an excessive amount of sugar. Be that as it may, anticipating the heightening of prediabetes into type 2 diabetes can be less difficult for a few.

Roughly 22 percent of individuals determined to have prediabetes can keep it from advancing to type 2 diabetes. One of the most significant factors in forestalling type 2 diabetes and bringing blood sugars once more into a more beneficial range comes down to grasping a plant-based diet.

"Plant-based dietary examples, particularly when they are improved with fortifying plant-based nourishments, might be valuable for the essential aversion of type 2 diabetes," clarified the report.

"Plant-based" is an in vogue term nowadays — and regularly suggests veganism — however in this unique circumstance, the focal point of a plant-put together diet is with respect to eating generally "genuine" nourishment, including some creature protein and carbohydrates.

Handled nourishments versus plant-based eating regimen

The most prompt advantage of a plant-put together diet with respect to the counteractive action of type 2 diabetes is the effect that non-plant-put together nourishments have with respect to glucose levels and insulin opposition.

As it is, look into recommends the effect is really more extensive.

"Plant-based eating regimens may likewise lessen the danger of type 2 diabetes through bringing down the danger of overabundance weight gain," the scientists noted.

"Different interventional and observational studies have demonstrated that expanded utilization of plant-based nourishments can prompt transient weight loss or counteractive action of long haul weight gain," clarified the specialists. "Thus, almost certainly, an extensive proportion of the defensive relationship between plant-based eating regimens and danger of type 2 diabetes can be owing to weight control."

Specialists in diabetes care and counteractive action concur.

"Imagine a scenario in which we had a world without handled nourishment in it?" We wouldn't have the weight issues we have now if not for prepared nourishment. It would be hard to get large while eating an entire nourishment, plant-based eating regimen."

Enjoying a pack of chips and a milkshake is significantly simpler than eating a bowl of custom made whipped cream with new blueberries and strawberries.

The distinction in results when a customer focuses on changing their sustenance propensities.

"Individuals really need to comprehend that what they put in their mouth influences their wellbeing," "You're going to need to focus on yourselves and recognize that your present eating routine is harming you."

The ongoing examination prescribes concentrating on a plant-based eating routine of fruits, vegetables, entire grains, vegetables, and nuts.

"In addition, refined grains, starches, and sugars can likewise be described as plant-based, despite the fact that they are autonomously connected with a higher danger of type 2 diabetes," the specialists said.

The investigation additionally found a "defensive" relationship against the improvement of type 2 diabetes when individuals devoured higher measures of nutrients, minerals, and cell reinforcements through plant nourishments and lower measures of red meats and handled meats.

The examination doesn't exhort against eating more beneficial creature items, for example, natural eggs, and lean proteins, similar to chicken, turkey, and pork.

It isn't simply insulin obstruction

"By eating an inappropriate nourishments, we increment our insulin levels," said Schwartz. "Expanded insulin levels really obstruct the generation of leptin."

Leptin is a lesser-examined however significant piece of dealing with your craving. It's a hormone created by your muscle to fat ratio's cells and your small digestion tracts. Its essential job is to direct your craving by motioning to your mind that you're full.

At the point when an individual creates "leptin opposition" from unnecessary measures of leptin in their framework alongside insulin obstruction, your cerebrum believes you're starving, making a voracious sort of yearning that prompts careless eating, needing low quality nourishment, and eating progressively prepared carbohydrates.

Turning around this beginnings with rolling out significant improvements in your eating routine by diminishing intensely prepared, bundled nourishments and concentrating each meal on entire food sources.

TIPS FOR PLANT-BASED DIET

There are a huge amount of disarrays about eating a plant-based eating schedule. I believe these tips can assist clear with increasing a portion of those confused decisions for plant-based students. As people grow progressively aware of their sustenance and lifestyle choices and veganism as a way of life is wrapping up progressively increasingly standard. Critical associations are watching, and the number and nature of vegan things at the business sectors are persistently extending. In the event that you're enthused about eating plant-based for your prosperity, the animals and the planet, this is the perfect chance to put everything hanging in the balance!

TIPS FOR EATING A PLANT-BASED DIET

1. Gradually and cautiously.

On the off chance that you're a plant-based amateur, upgrading your eating routine likely won't happen with no thinking ahead. It will require some venture to become adjusted to, and there's nothing not right with a moderate change.

WHERE TO START

Have a go toward the start with 1-2 meatless days out of every week, by then extending that as you get logically okay with plant-based eating. Next, start overriding the dairy in your eating schedule. This is more straightforward than you may speculate. Approach things gradually and cautiously. Start by supplanting the cream in your coffee with your most cherished non-dairy milk by then diminish or take out cheddar by getting some answers concerning vegan decisions. At the point when you have a hold on living sans dairy, it's a superb chance to deal with eggs. Eggs are definitely not hard to replace in your eating schedule, don't eat them.

This being expressed, if it's not all that much issue note tip #2. If you wind up falling back on animal things over and over, at any rate, endeavor to diminish the proportion of meat, dairy and eggs you exhaust. I would want to see you find something achievable than give up completely. I've been eating thusly a long time, and it as a rule comes to me now. The best movement starts every meal thusly. Definitely it will end up being normal.

2. Cast off RULES AND LABELS.

At the point when you're only start, it will put aside some push to adapt to not eating and cooking with animal things.

It gets less complex, sticks to it keep learning, and over the long haul, it will be hard to envision eating and cooking with meat and dairy things. I confide in it's your primary concern dependably as time goes on that has a noteworthy impact, so on the off chance that you eat a pinch of cheddar or a thing that contains milk, don't pound yourself, life is unreasonably short. Continue ahead and come back to common.

VOTE WITH YOUR DOLLARS

Another brilliant starting stage is just monitoring where you spend your dollars. Reinforce close by sustenance providers where possible and don't buy mass-conveyed, modern office developed animal things. We eat in any occasion multiple times every day, and every meal is a chance to either hit a homerun bat for having confidence in or continue supporting what you don't, to support your body with whole, stable sustenance or do the opposite. Pick cautiously.

3. KEEP IN YOUR WHY.

For what reason did you live without animal things in your eating schedule? Did you see a plant developing video that affected you? Did you read a book that changed how you think about our sustenance system and how we treat animals? Is it cautiously for your prosperity? Constantly profit to that why for the off possibility that you wind up endeavoring to keep up a strong, plant-based eating routine.

TRANSITION TO A PLANT-BASED DIET

In case you've been eating a seriously animal based eating routine, the change to a plant-based eating routine may have all the earmarks of being boundless. You may make sense of what one may have the option to eat, maybe in the event that you don't eat meat, eggs and dairy? Don't you stress? I'm here to ensure that not only is there a ton of supporting, delicious sustenances to eat; in any case, they can be prepared as fun and creative plant-based choices rather than all your favored nourishment sources.

CHANGING YOUR MINDSET

It's fundamental to move toward this new part with an open viewpoint and a rousing frame of mind. Endeavor to think with respect to what you'll be getting from eating a plant-based eating routine as opposed to what you'll be leaving behind. Keeping up your new diet shouldn't be about self-control, fight or hardship. Believe it or not, when you get acquainted with plant-based eating, you'll see that don't have to give up anything. At the point when you're OK with the complex subtleties of vegan alternatives as opposed to pizza, treats, bread rolls, chocolate and sandwiches, you'll have no issue making sense of how to treasure the plant-based lifestyle and how it influences you.

KNOW YOUR REASON WHY

It's basic to get genuinely clear on your motivation behind setting out on a whole sustenance plant-based) diet. On the off chance that it's a critical lifestyle change for you, it will get exceptional now and again and having an unquestionable inspiration driving for what reason can empower you to cling to your targets.

Clarifications behind eating plant-based could include:

• counteracting disease

• Managing glucose

• bringing down cholesterol

• living longer

• love for animals

• shedding pounds

• decreasing your normal impact

There are a huge amount of exceptional inspirations to eat a plant-based eating routine. What one tends to you?

Find a clarification that rouses and empowers you and get really clear on it. Record your why and stick it on your cooler or washroom reflect. Keep that reason forthright to empower you to stay focused.

WHAT IS A WHOLE FOOD PLANT-BASED DIET?

An entire eating regimen means eating complete, foul or negligibly handled plant nourishments. It depends on organic products, vegetables, tubers, whole grains, vegetables, nuts and seeds. Being plant-based, it rejects meat, dairy items, eggs and refined grains, sugars and oil.

WHAT'S THE DIFFERENCE BETWEEN PLANT-BASED AND VEGAN

We should talk a tad about the contrast between vegan and plant-based. While they're fundamentally the same as you might be vegan yet not eat an entire nourishment plant-based eating routine or you may eat a plant-based eating routine however not be vegan.

Veganism is the act of limiting mischief to all creatures by swearing off creature items, for example, meat, fish, dairy, eggs, nectar, gelatin, lanolin, fleece, hide, silk, softened cowhide, and calfskin. It is more than an eating routine, and it is a method for living that tries to reject all types of abuse and cold-bloodedness to creatures for nourishment, attire or some other reason.

To be vegan, it would mean no down sofa-beds, no fleece socks, no nectar, no gelatin-based treats and obviously, no eating dairy, eggs, meat or fish.

A plant-put together diet concerning the next hand is just about the nourishment. You can think about what it's about from the name. On the off chance that you eat a plant-based eating regimen, you may not be vegan, and you may have different purposes behind eating that route than just empathy.

WHAT'S THE DIFFERENCE BETWEEN A VEGAN AND VEGETARIAN DIET?

Vegetarians don't eat creatures, for example, cows, pigs or fish yet at the same time incorporate creature items, for example, dairy and eggs in their eating regimen. Vegans don't eat or utilize any creature items. That implies no meat, fish, eggs or dairy.

PLANT-BASED VS WHOLE FOOD PLANT-BASED
A plant-based or vegan diet could be comprised of prepared nourishment, sugars, refined grains and undesirable fats, that is the place whole nourishment plant-based comes in. An entire nourishment plant-based intends to limit or wipe out prepared nourishments and stick to nourishments as near their natural state as could reasonably be expected.

WHY WHOLE FOOD PLANT-BASED?
By eating grungy nourishments, we can exploit all the large scale and micronutrients we need yet none of the garbage we don't. Diminishing refined sugars, grains and oils are significant in decreasing aggravation.

TIPS BEFORE STARTING YOUR PLANT-BASED JOURNEY
There are a couple of parts of proper dieting that I see as key to progress. Audit these tips before you begin.

PREPARE YOUR FOOD.
This is likely the most significant part of eating plant-based. Except if you have tremendous assets for nourishment and live someplace with vast amounts of vegan eateries, preparing your food at home is entirely crucial to making an entire nourishment plant-based eating regimen work. So it's an ideal opportunity to get in the kitchen! There's no compelling reason to go through hours cooking, making healthy plant-based meals can be brisk and basic.

MEAL PLAN AND FOOD PREP.
I prescribe doing probably some nourishment prep consistently. It will make your life so a lot simpler, set aside your cash and avoid nourishment squander. I would likewise suggest plunking down on Sundays and finishing a meal plan and staple rundown: arranging and preparation and the key to progress.
When you have an arrangement for the week and an entire basic food item show, it's an excellent opportunity to shop and after that get in the kitchen to do some nourishment prep. This could be a basic as pre-washing and hacking every one of your veggies, or as careful as clump preparing every one of your meals for the week. Trial and see what works for you.

STOCK YOUR PANTRY.
Having a well-loaded washroom of basics will rearrange your shopping records and enable you to make substantial and tasty meals on the fly.

TEACH YOURSELF.
This progression is enormous, as well. All the more you find out about wellbeing, sustenance, creature welfare and farming, the simpler settling on plant-based decisions progresses toward becoming.

PROGRESS NOT PERFECTION.

This is so significant, and I see it over and over, individuals have one setback and after that surrender totally. This is in reverse reasoning. It resembles dropping your PDA and after that crushing it totally, or getting a gap in one tire and supplanting every one of the four with new ones. Staggering is no major ordeal, and the key is to lift yourself back up and continue pushing ahead. Never discard all your diligent work due to one little disappointment. Disappointment is how we learn and develop. Consistency is unquestionably more significant than flawlessness. Flawlessness doesn't exist at all, so be thinking to yourself, excuse yourself, perceive progress huge or little and continue onward. We're all human.

CONCLUSION

Instead of what different people may think, sound plant based recipes are not exactly as of late simple to make yet rather are also great and more than pleasing. Every vegetable has a specific flavor inside, and when solidified, vegetables can convey a taste that will place cheeseburger and pork recipes into disfavor. The best error with vegetarian recipes is that since the Food doesn't have any meat on the fixing' lists, it will normally taste dull and debilitating. That is the reason meat darlings simply show that the vegetarian recipes are not excessively much delectable and heavenly as meat recipes.